UNDERGRADUATE ORTHOPAEDIC HISTORY AND PHYSICAL EXAMINATION TECHNIQUES

Biju Benjamin
MBBS, MS (Tr & Ortho), MCh (Tr & Ortho), MFSEM (Ireland), Fellow AANOS (US)
Associate Professor, Royal College of Medicine Perak, University of Kuala Lumpur, Malaysia

CONTENTS

PREFACE

While conducting classes and bed side sessions for undergraduate medical students during their orthopaedic posting, it is often noticed that history taking and clinical examination of patients can be a daunting task for students. Students are often confused regarding the myriad of tests and examination techniques described in the various available textbooks. Hence it was planned to make available a book for easy reading and understanding with diagrammatic representation of the various tests. With the popularity and easy usage of electronic media, this book is being made available in E-book format.

The first edition of this E-book is mainly intended to appeal to undergraduate medical students and residents in their early years of training. Although a great deal of experience is required to take an adequate history and do a thorough examination, it is hoped that this book provides the necessary knowledge and confidence to ensure that the process will be smooth.

ACKNOWLEDGEMENTS

I' am grateful to the University of Kuala Lumpur, Malaysia for providing me the opportunity to author this E-book. I' am also grateful to my colleagues in my department for encouraging me in this endeavor.

My biggest thanks is to my wife Mridula and daughter Alyssa who allowed me enough time to put this book together.

PRELIMINARY REQUIREMENTS

- Introduce yourself to the patient and explain your role.
- Confirm identity of patient.
- Adequate history should be obtained.
- Ensure privacy for the patient.
- Ensure chaperone before examination.
- Gather all necessary equipment before commencing examination.
- Equipment required include, stethoscope, thermometer, sphygmomanometer, penlight, tape measure, watch, pen, cotton, pin and assessment notes paper.
- Ensure the modesty of patient at all times, but adequate exposure is essential.
- Wash your hands before and after examination.
- If contamination of body fluids is anticipated, don personal protective equipment (PPE) such as gloves, mask and disposable apron.
- Once you complete the examination, dispose the PPE safely.
- Thank the patient before leaving the room.

HISTORY TAKING

History taking is the most important step in making a diagnosis. A clinician is 60% closer to making a diagnosis with a thorough history. The remaining 40% is a combination of examination findings and investigations.
- Develop rapport with the patient.
- Make patient comfortable.
- Be well composed, confident, well dressed and not in a hurry.
- Listen to patient but do not get carried away.
- Intelligent cross questioning.
- Document legibly with no abbreviations.

PATIENT DETAILS

- Name, age, sex, address.
- Date of history taking.
- Informant of the history.

PRESENTING COMPLAINTS

- In the words of the patient.
- Should be the complaint that has brought the patient to the hospital.
- Must mention the duration of symptoms and mechanism of onset.
- If more than one complaint mention them in chronological order.
- If few complaints have started at same time, list them in order of severity.

Eg. Pain right thigh following alleged road traffic accident 3 days ago.

HISTORY OF PRESENTING COMPLAINTS

- Onset of symptoms: Trauma / non-trauma. If alleged trauma, explain the mechanism of trauma in detail.
- Explain the presenting complaint in detail including the progression of the condition.

Pain
- Site.
- Onset/duration.
- Type of pain: Sharp/throbbing/dull/shooting.
- Radiation of pain.
- Intensity of pain.
- Degree of disability.
- Aggravating and alleviating factors.
- Associated symptoms.

Swelling
- Site.
- Duration.
- Local vs. generalized.
- Onset.
- Constant or off and on.
- Progression: Same size or increasing. If increasing, rapidly or slowly.
- Aggravating and relieving factors.
- Associated with injury or reactive.
- Painful or not.

Instability
- Onset.
- How did it start?
- Any history of trauma?
- Frequency.
- Trigger/aggravating factors.
- Does the joint lock?
- Does the joint click or clunk?
-         Associated symptoms: Swelling, pain.

Deformity
- Duration.
- Progressive or not?
- Associated with symptoms like pain & stiffness.
- Impaired function or not?

Limping
- Painful vs. painless.
- Onset (acute or chronic).
- Progressive or not?
- Use of walking aid.
- Functional disability?
- Traumatic or non-traumatic.
- Associated with swelling, deformity, or fever.

Loss of function
- How has this affected life?
- Is it interfering with activities of daily living (ADL), work or sport?

Stiffness
- Onset of stiffness.
- Progression of stiffness.
- Affecting activities of daily living?

PAST HISTORY

- Any previous injuries.
- Any previous surgeries.
- Relevant past disease: Diabetes, hypertension, tuberculosis, asthma.

DRUG HISTORY, PERSONAL, OCCUPATIONAL, SOCIAL & FAMILY HISTORY

- Mention all the medications the patient is currently taking.
- Children should be asked about immunization history.
- Occupation.
- Living style.
- Smoking/drinking: Quantity.
- In women, menstrual history should be taken.
- Relevant family history for any genetic link to disease.

RED FLAGS IN HISTORY

- Pain at night or rest.
- Thoracic pain.
- Associated weight loss and loss of appetite.
- Fever/night sweats.
- Fever ≥38°C for 48 hours.
- History of cancer.
- Steroid use.
- History of trauma.
- Extremes of age.
- Bowel or bladder symptoms.
- Saddle numbness or anaesthesia.

YELLOW FLAGS IN HISTORY

- A belief that the pain is harmful or potentially disabling.
- Fear, avoidance behavior and reduced activity levels.
- Tendency to low mood and withdrawal from social interaction.
- Expectation of passive treatments rather than a belief that active participation will help.
- Problems with claims and compensation.
- Past history of back pain, time-off and other claims.
- Problems at work, poor job satisfaction, heavy work and unsociable hours.
- Overprotective family or lack of support.

GENERAL EXAMINATION

- Level of consciousness and orientation:
    - Is he awake and alert?
    - Is he oriented to PERSON: Knows his name?
    - Is he oriented to PLACE: KNOWS where he is?
    - Is he oriented to TIME: Knows the day and date?
- Attitude of the patient.
- Head: Shape and symmetry; condition of hair and scalp.
- Eyes: Conjunctiva and sclera for anaemia and jaundice. Pupils: reactivity to light and ability to follow your finger or a light.
- Ears: Hearing aids, pain, bleeding?
- Nose: Difficulty breathing, bleeding?
- Throat and mouth: Mucous membranes, any lesions, teeth or dentures, swallowing, trachea, lymph nodes, tongue, bleeding.
- Neck: Obvious swellings, neck tenderness.
- Chest: Chest compression for tenderness, air entry, heart sounds.
- Abdomen: Soft, tenderness, bowel sounds, palpate the bladder.
- Pelvis: Pelvic compression test.
- Upper limbs: Capillary refill, clubbing, temperature, ROM. Palpate for pulses.
- Lower limbs: Temperature, capillary fill, pedal edema and ROM. Palpate for pulses.
- Vital signs:
    Pulse.
    Blood pressure.
    Respiratory rate.
    Temperature.

EXAMINATION OF SUSPECTED FRACTURES

INSPECTION

- Abnormal swelling.
- Deformity.
- Attitude of limb.
- Shortening.
- Overlying skin: Wounds, blisters, abrasions or bruising.

PALPATION

- Bony tenderness.
- Bone irregularity.
- Abnormal mobility: Useful to assess non-union and not in acute fractures
- Crepitus: Should be never elicited.
- Examination of swelling.
- Examination of any wounds: Assess size of wound, contamination and active bleeding.
- Check for distal pulses, capillary refill and sensations.

MOVEMENTS

- Both active and passive movements of the involved area. But this is not done if an acute fracture is confirmed.
- Examine movements of the distal parts of the limb to rule out any nerve injuries.

MEASUREMENT

- Length: To rule out shortening. Compare with opposite limb after placing both limbs in identical position.
- Circumference: To look for complications like compartment syndrome and muscle wasting in late cases.
    Always measure the healthy limb first.
    Measurements should be made at the same level in both limbs. So use a bony landmark as reference point.

CHECK FOR ASSOCIATED INJURIES

- Vital signs.
- Nerves, vessels.
- Head injury.
- Internal organs of thorax, abdomen and pelvis.

EXAMINATION OF SHOULDER

ANATOMY

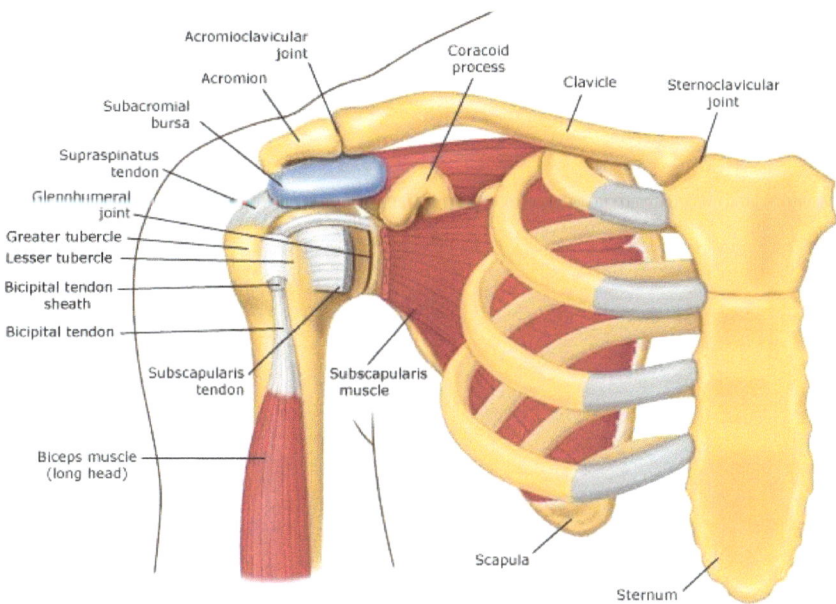

Fig. 1: Anterior view

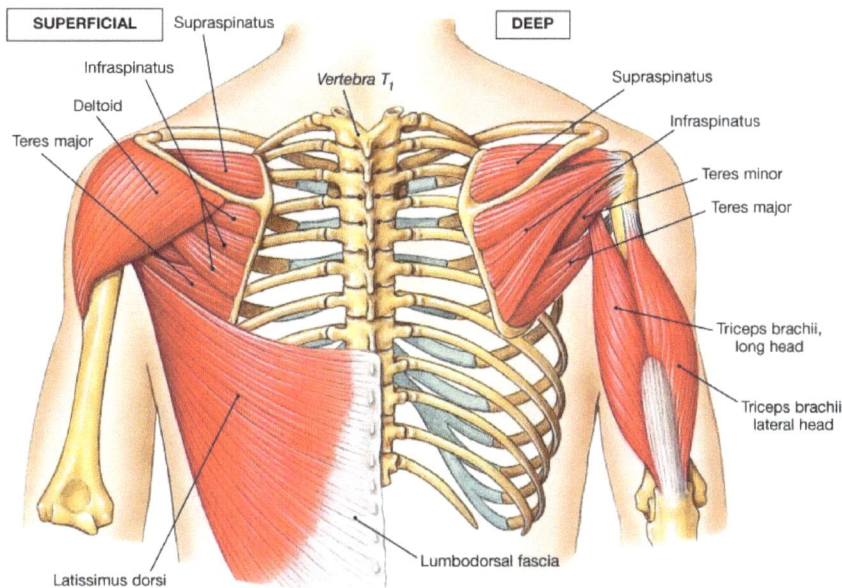

Fig. 2: Posterior view

INSPECTION

Make sure the patient is adequately exposed to view the shoulder from both the front and the back. Compare both shoulders, and have a good look around from all angles.

- Skin colour changes.
- Bruising, external injuries.
- Scars.
- Wasting:
    Wasting at the side: Deltoid muscle. This could cause the shoulder to become flattened. Often secondary to nerve lesion.
    Wasting at the back: Trapezius muscle.
- Deformity.
    Squaring of shoulder: Seen in shoulder dislocation. (Fig. 1)
    Deformity over the clavicle or AC joint: suggests previous fracture or AC dislocation. (Fig. 2)
    Generalized swelling: probably caused by effusion.
    Popeye sign: Flex the arm at the elbow to look for ruptured biceps tendon. You will see a large mass of muscle either near the elbow joint, or anywhere further up the humerus. (Fig. 3)
    Winging of scapula: Ask the patient to push against a wall. The scapula becomes abnormally laterally rotated. It is due to a lesion of the long thoracic nerve resulting in serratus anterior paralysis. (Fig. 4)

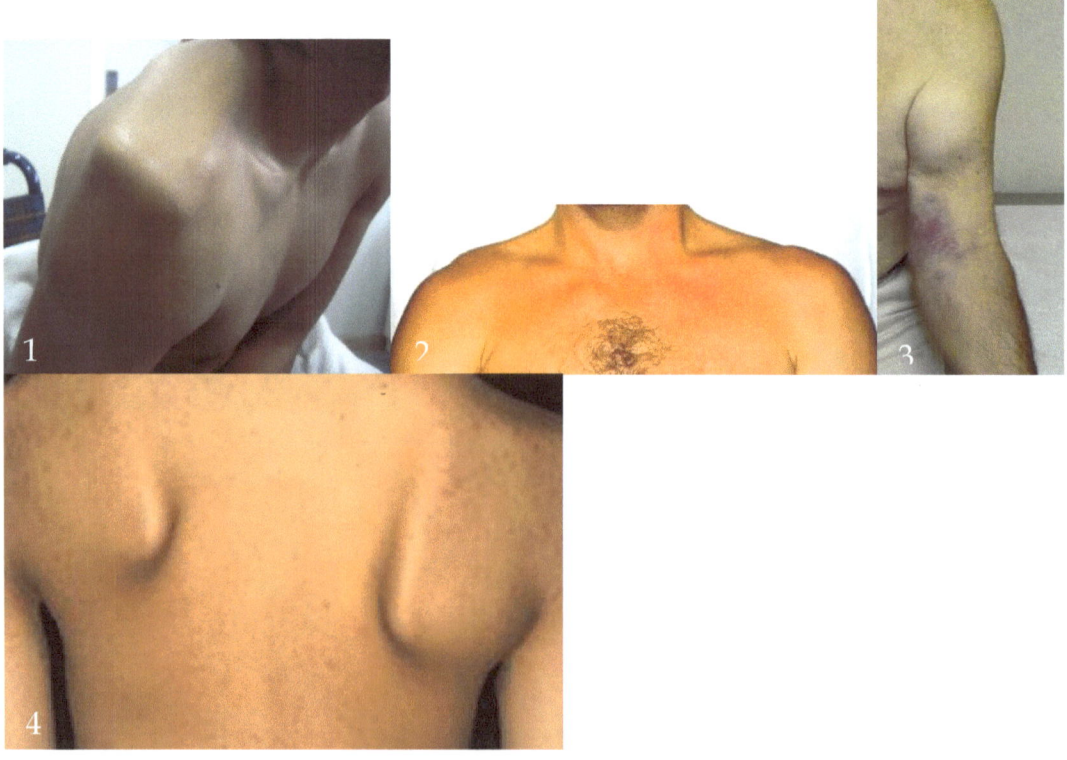

PALPATION

Ask the patient if they have any pain before you start palpating. As you palpate, look at the patients face to see if you elicit any pain.

- Palpate for tenderness and temperature changes.
- Start at the sternum, sternoclavicular joint and move laterally along the clavicle, until you reach the acromio-clavicular joint. Feel this joint, then move along and feel along the spine of the scapula. Then feel the greater tuberosity, the anterior and posterior joint lines of the gleno-humeral joint and for general muscle tenderness.
- While palpating also feel for any crepitus. This is a crunching, grating feeling inside the joint, indicative of degeneration. If crepitus is felt along bone, it could indicate a fracture.
- Palpation of the dorsal spine and inter-scapular area: this area is sometimes called a trigger point for fibromyalgia. (Fig. 1) Palpating this area in individuals with this condition can elicit pain.

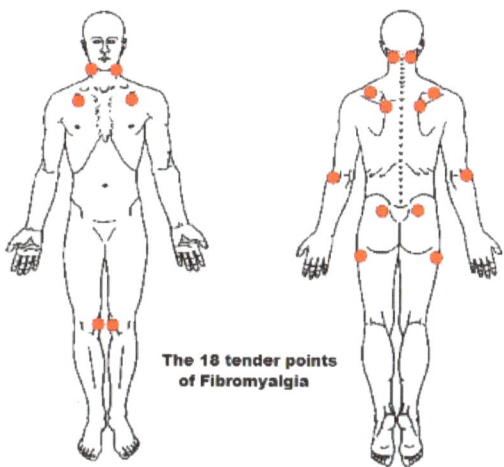

The 18 tender points
of Fibromyalgia

MOVEMENTS

Begin with active movements, followed by passive movements. (Fig. 1)

- Abduction: 0-150 degrees.
- Adduction: 0-45 degrees.
- Flexion: 0-180 degrees.
- Extension: 45-60 degrees.
- Internal rotation: test with elbow flexed to 90 degrees. 70-90 degrees.
- External rotation: test with elbow flexed to 90 degrees. 0-90 degrees.
  Can also be tested by the Apley scratch test: Ask patient to put the backs of their hands on their bottom. How high up their back can they reach? Normal is about L4. If they cannot get up very high, external rotation may be reduced. (Fig. 2)

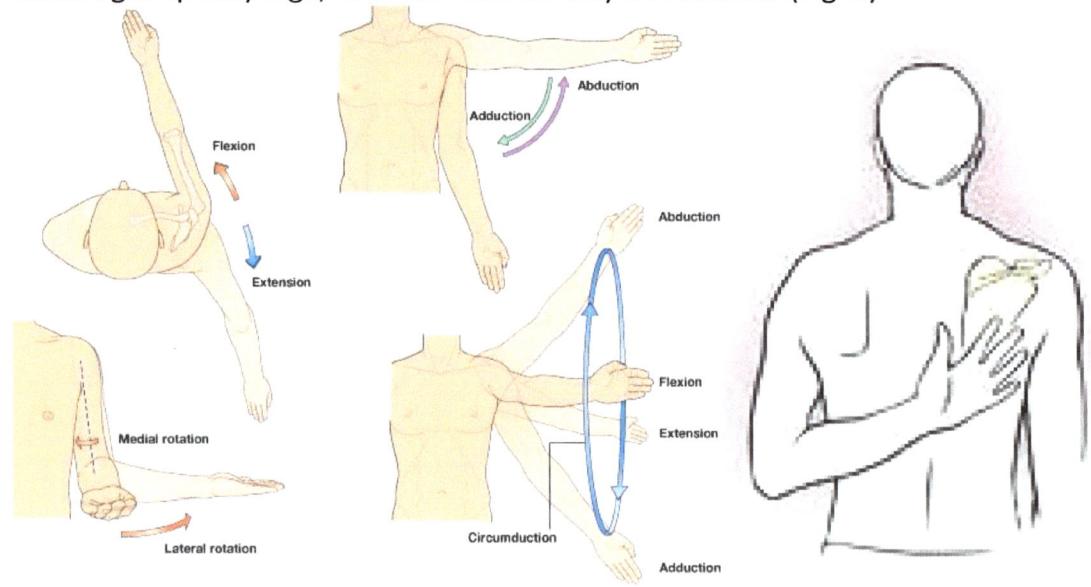

<u>SPECIAL TESTS</u>

- Rotator cuff muscle power testing
    1. Supraspinatus: can be assessed using 2 tests.
        a. Empty can/Jobes's test: The patient's arm is abducted to 90 degrees and brought forward to about 30 degrees. Elbow is fully extended and full pronation of the forearm is maintained. This results in a thumbs-down position, as if the patient were pouring liquid out of a can. Apply a downward directed force to the arm and the patient tries to resist this motion. This test is considered positive if the patient experiences pain or weakness with resistance. (Fig. 1)
        b. Drop arm test: Stand behind the seated patient and abduct patient's arm to 90^0, supporting the arm at the elbow. Release the elbow support, and ask patient to slowly lower the arm to the side. Test is positive if there is pain while lowering the arm, sudden dropping of the arm or weakness in maintaining arm position during lowering, suggesting injury to the supraspinatus. (Fig. 2)
    2. Infraspinatus / teres minor: Elbow tucked into chest well, flexed at 90 degrees. Patient tries to move palms apart (external rotation) against resistance. (Fig. 3)
    3. Subscapularis: can be assessed using 2 tests.
        a. Gerber's lift off test: The patient is examined in standing and is asked to place their hand behind their back with the dorsum of the hand resting in the region of the mid- lumbar spine. Patient is asked to actively lift the dorsum of the hand off the back with the examiner resisting it. Inability to move the dorsum off the back constitutes an abnormal lift-off test and indicates subscapularis rupture or dysfunction. (Fig. 4)
        b. Belly press test: The patients hand is placed flat on their abdomen. The patient is then instructed to press down on the abdomen and the examiner tries to pull the hand away from the abdomen. A positive test is an inability to compresses the abdomen without flexing at the wrist (Fig. 5)

- Test for shoulder impingement:
    a. Hawkin's test: Ask the patient to flex their shoulder to 90 degrees. Then flex the elbow to 90 degrees so that this forearm is parallel to the floor. Support the elbow and press down on the patient's wrist. This movement forcibly rotates the shoulder joint internally. This is a passive movement, so the patient should be relaxed. This basically presses the tendons of the shoulder cuff against the coraco-humeral ligament. A positive test is when pain is elicited. (Fig. 6)
    b. Painful arc: With the patient in either sitting or standing the patient should be instructed to abduct the arm. While abducting the arm, if the patient experiences any pain in and around the gleno-humeral joint the patient must tell it to the examiner. The patient is instructed to continue abducting the arm as high as they

can. One the patient gets to approximately 120 degrees of abduction there should be a reduction in the amount of pain being experienced. Following completion of the abduction movement the patient should then slowly reverse the motion, bring the arm back to neutral position via the movement of adduction. This test is considered to be positive if the patient experiences pain between 40 and 120 degrees of abduction which reduces once past 120 degrees of abduction. (Fig. 7)

- Apprehension test: This is so called because it asks if the patient is 'apprehensive' about certain shoulder movements – i.e. they feel their shoulder joint is unstable in some positions. Ask the patient to externally rotate and abduct the shoulder, whilst also flexing the elbow. Then place your hand on the patient's wrist, and your other hand near the head of the humerus, on the posterior surface of the arm. Try to push the humerus forward against the shoulder joint. If this elicits discomfort, it is a positive apprehension test. (Fig. 8)

- Dugas test: With the patient seated, instruct to place hand on opposite shoulder and touch elbow to chest. Pain & inability to perform indicates dislocation of shoulder. (Fig. 9)

- Test for Biceps tendon: 2 tests.
  a. Speed's test: Patent is seated with straight arm and shoulder flexed to 90 degrees and forearm fully supinated. Patient is now asked to flex elbow with examiner resisting. Inability and pain is positive test. (Fig. 10)
  b. Yergason's test: The patient's elbow is flexed and their forearm pronated. The examiner holds their arm at the wrist. Patient actively supinates against resistance. Pain located to bicipital groove area suggests pathology in the long head of biceps. (Fig. 11)

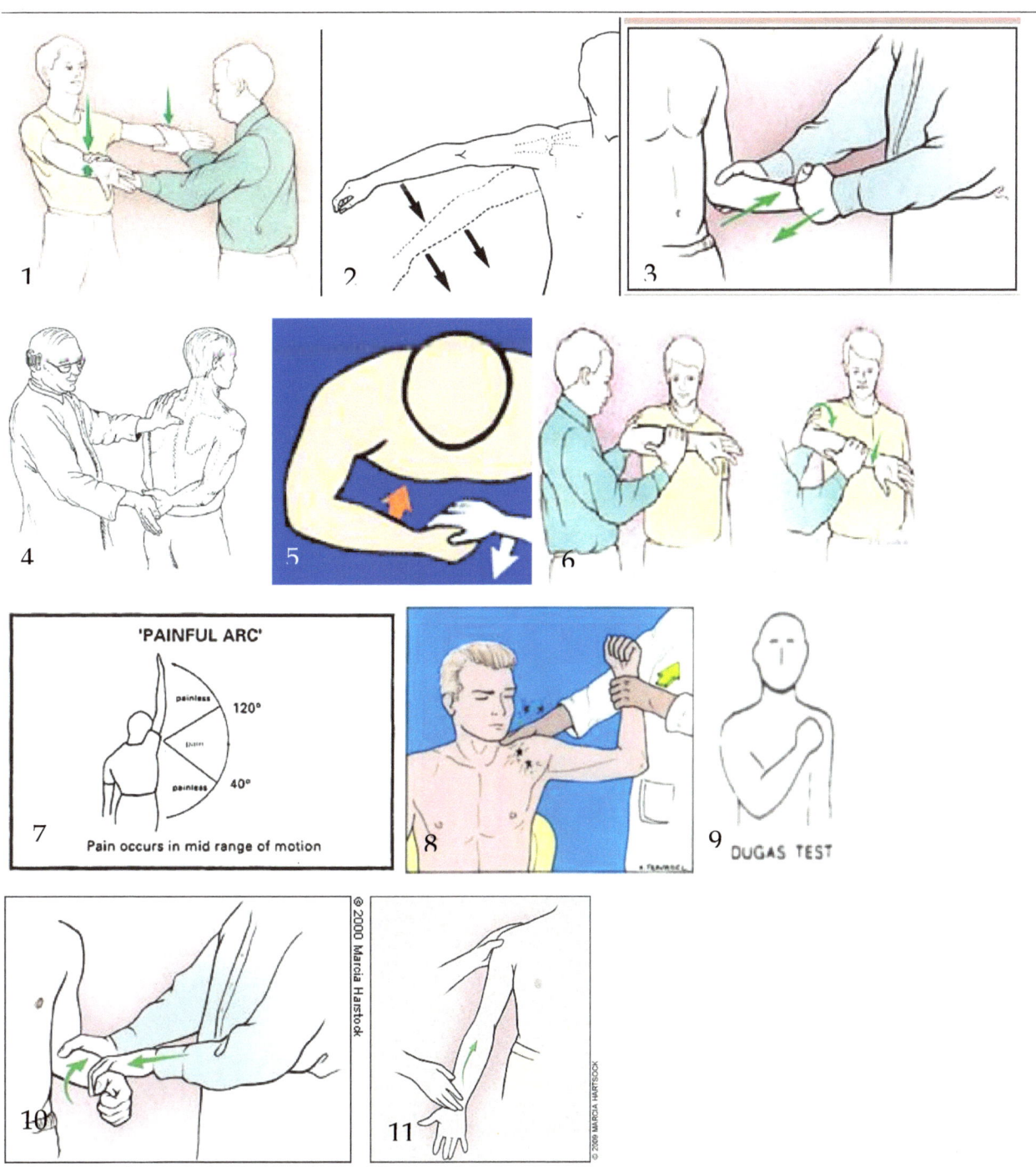

'PAINFUL ARC'

painless

120°

pain

painless

40°

Pain occurs in mid range of motion

DUGAS TEST

© 2000 Marcia Hartsook

© 2009 MARCIA HARTSOOK

EXAMINATION OF ELBOW

ANATOMY

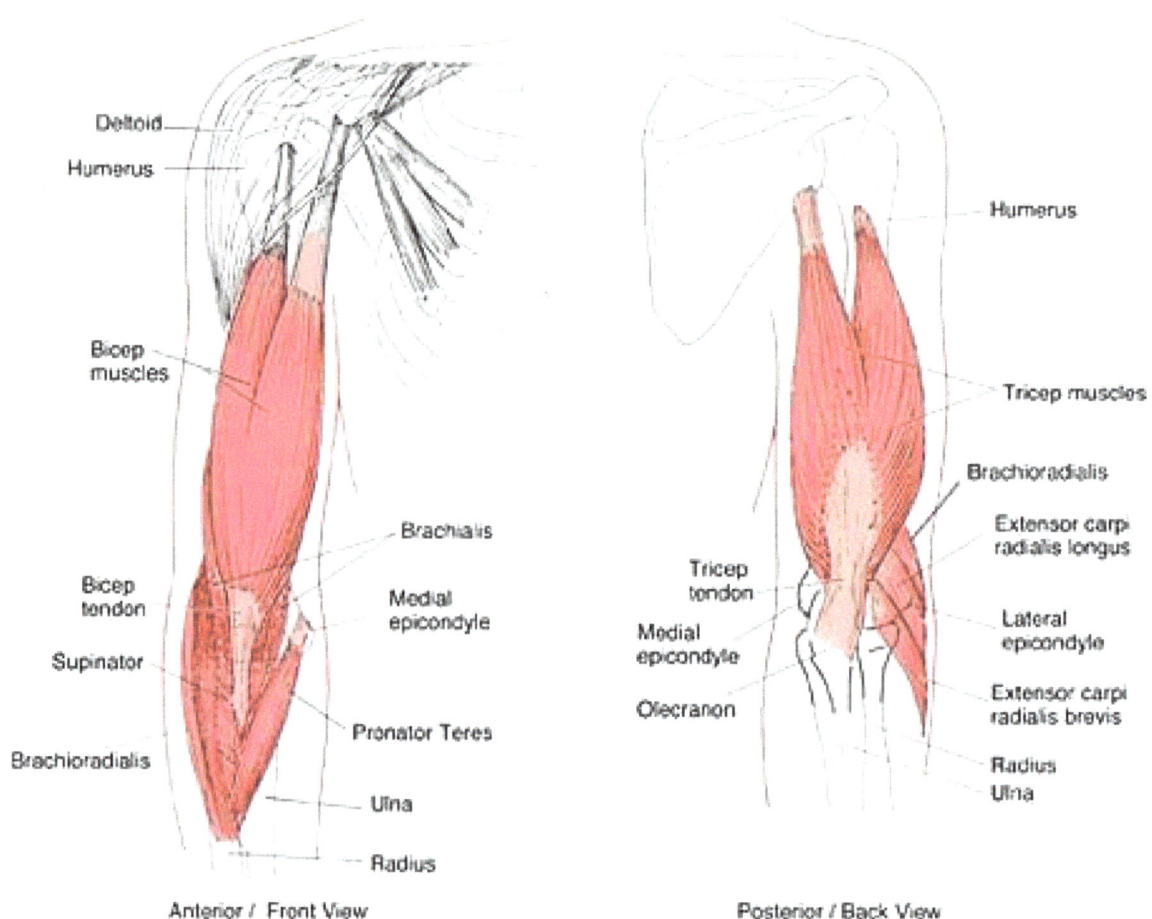

Anterior / Front View

Posterior / Back View

INSPECTION

- Look from the front for the carrying angle (Fig. 1), any varus / gun-stock deformity (Fig. 2) and from the side for flexion deformity.
- Look at elbow for scars, rashes, muscle wasting, rheumatoid nodules (Fig. 3), swellings and psoriatic plaques.

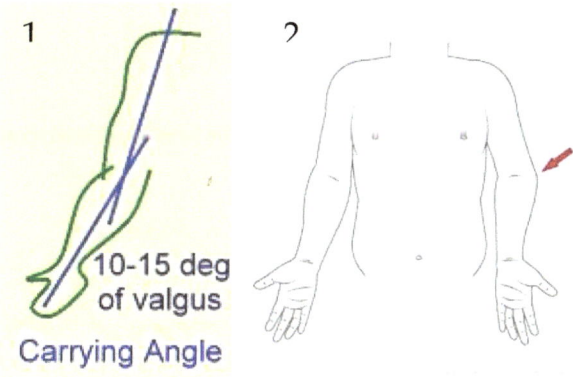

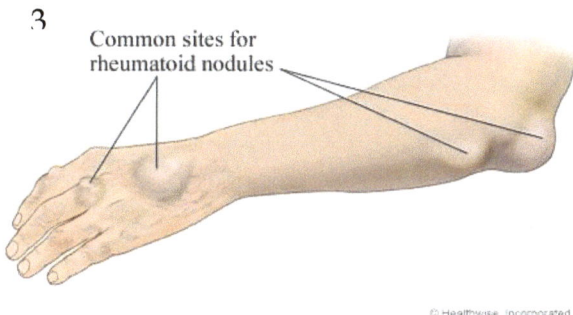

PALPATION

- Using the back of your hand, feel the temperature across the joint and the forearm.
- Holding the arm with one hand, palpate the elbow feeling for the joint line, checking for swelling, looking at patient's face for evidence of tenderness.
- Palpate the olecranon process for tenderness and evidence of bursitis.
- Palpate the medial epicondyle (golfer's elbow) and the lateral epicondyle (tennis elbow).

MOVEMENTS

- Actively before passively.
- Test extension and flexion – compare both sides with one another. 0-145 degrees. (Fig. 1)
- Assess pronation and supination. Feel for crepitus when moving passively. 70 degrees & 85 degrees. (Fig. 2)

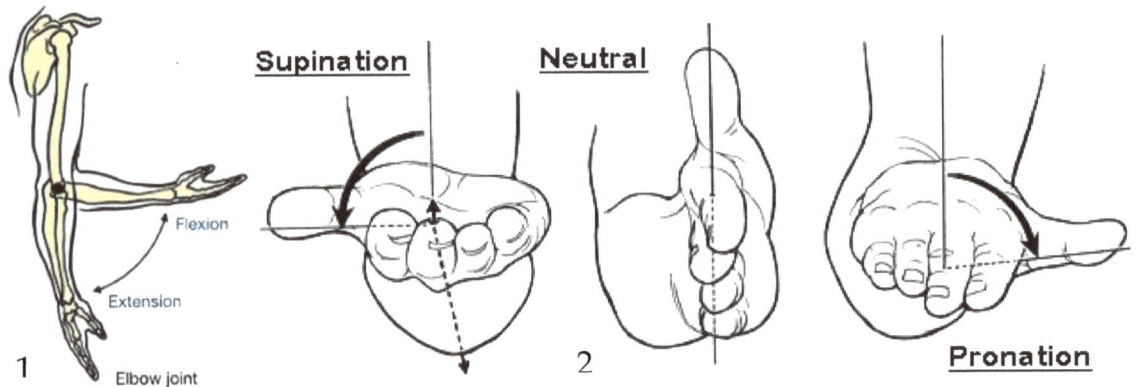

SPECIAL TESTS

- Golfer's elbow (medial epicondylitis): Check for tenderness over the medial epicondyle, and then ask the patient to hold out their arms in a pronated position, and make a fist. Flex the wrist against resistance. In cases of golfer's elbow, the pain will be worse on wrist flexion. (Fig. 1)
- Tennis elbow (lateral epicondylitis): Check if pain is worse on extension of the wrist. (Fig. 2)

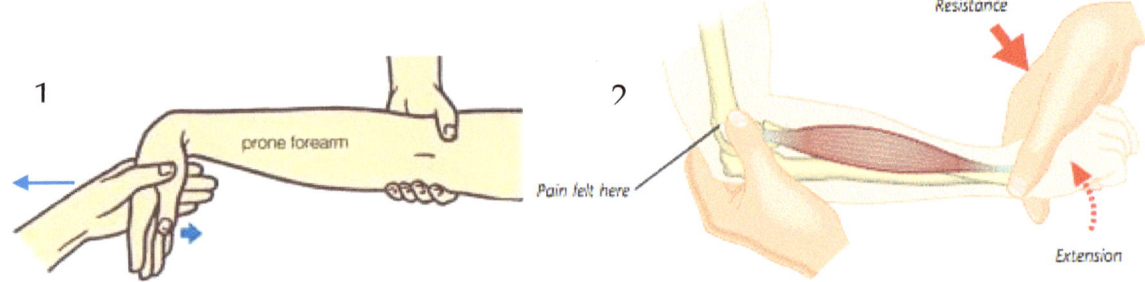

EXAMINATION OF WRIST

ANATOMY

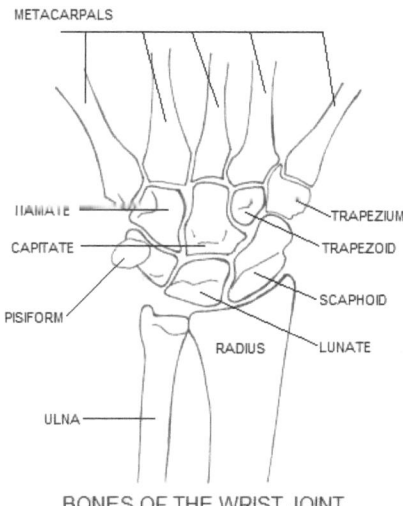

BONES OF THE WRIST JOINT

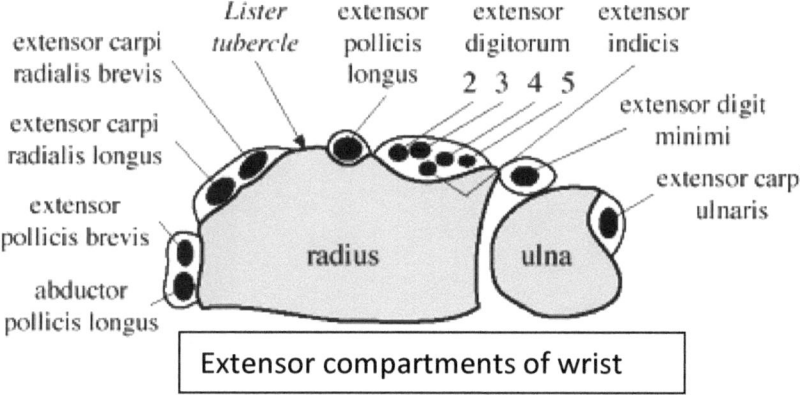

Extensor compartments of wrist

INSPECTION

Look at wrist for scars, rashes, muscle wasting, swellings and deformities.

PALPATION

Palpate bony points for tenderness. Also palpate the anatomical snuff box in suspected scaphoid fractures. Also palpate for any temperature changes and swellings.

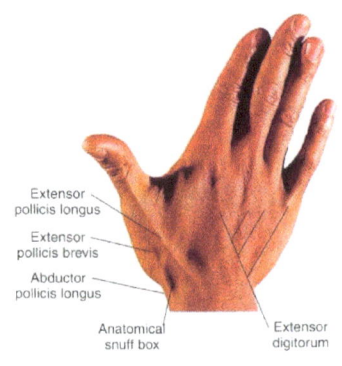

MOVEMENTS

Flexion: 75 degrees
Extension: 70 degrees
Radial deviation: 20 degrees
Ulnar deviation: 35 degrees

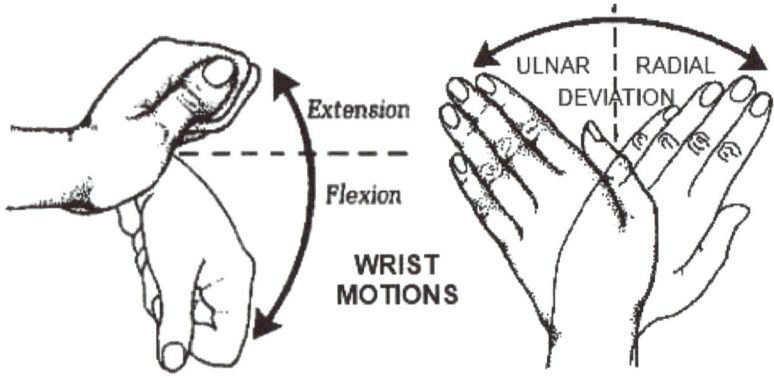

<u>SPECIAL TESTS</u>

Finkelstein's test: Used in the diagnosis of De Quervain's syndrome. Ask the patient to make a fist around a thumb and to perform an ulnar deviation. If the patient feels pain radiating up the inside of his or her arm from the thumb, the test is positive.

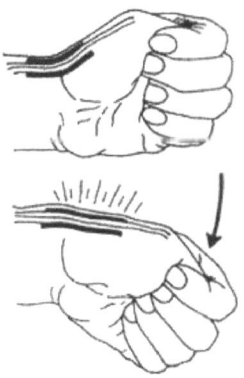

EXAMINATION OF HAND

ANATOMY

Bones of human hand and wrist

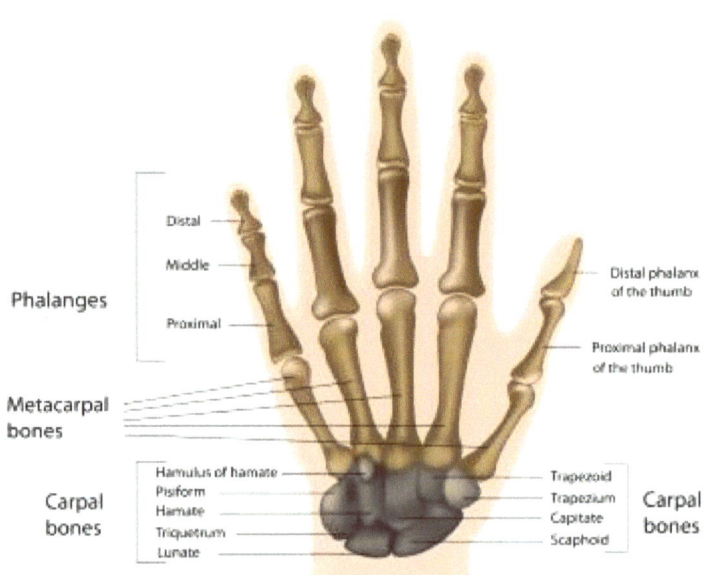

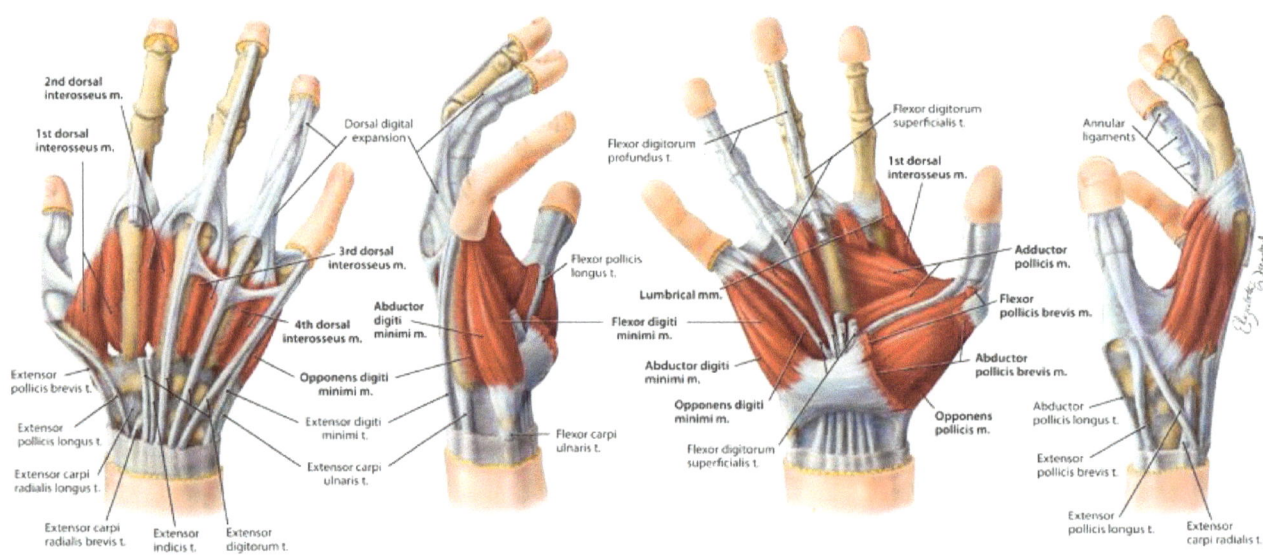

INSPECTION

Look for muscle wasting and any deformities such as wrist drop (Fig. 1) or claw hand (Fig. 2).
Look at the nails for pitting, splitting, onycholysis (Painless separation of the nail from the nail bed): Seen in psoriatic arthropathy (Fig. 3).
Longitudinal ridging of nails seen in Rheumatoid arthritis (Fig. 4).
Raynaud's phenomenon: White fingers when cold, become blue as they warm (Fig. 5).
Look for any rheumatoid nodules or gouty tophi (Fig. 6).
Look at the DIP and PIP for Heberden and Bouchard nodes (Fig. 7), swan neck deformity and Boutonniere deformity and mallet fingers (Fig. 8).

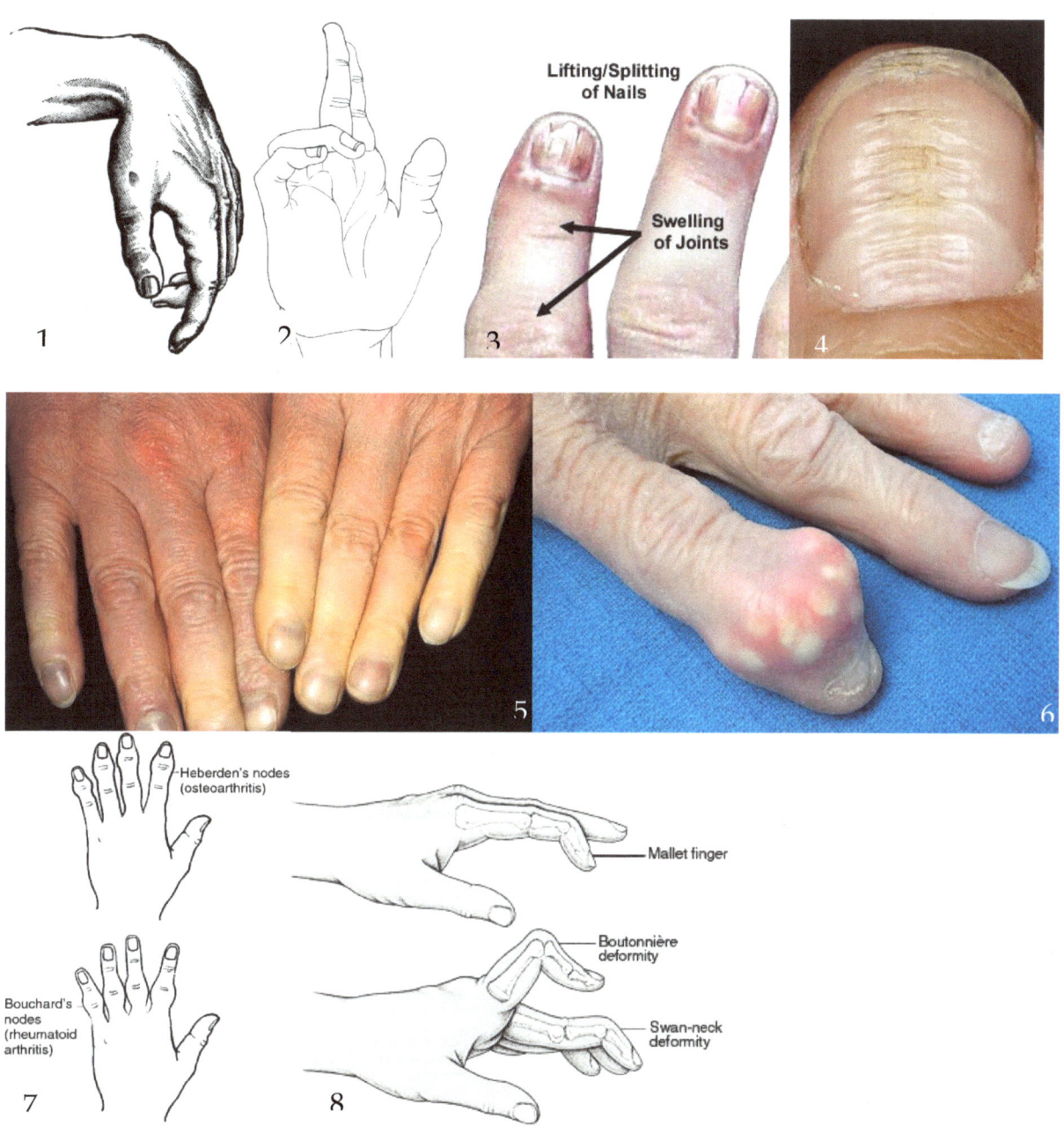

<u>PALPATION</u>

Feel the hand for any local tenderness and rise in temperature.

Assess any swelling if present.

Feel the MCP, PIP & DIP joints for dislocations and subluxations: relatively common in RA (Fig. 1).

Look and feel for muscle wasting:

- Diffuse atrophy: general wasting of the muscles of the hand. Probably as a result of disuse of the hand due to joint stiffness and pain.
- Median nerve lesion: wasting of the thenar eminence (Fig. 2).
- Ulnar nerve lesion pattern: wasting of the hypothenar eminence (Fig. 3) and interosseous muscles (Fig. 4).

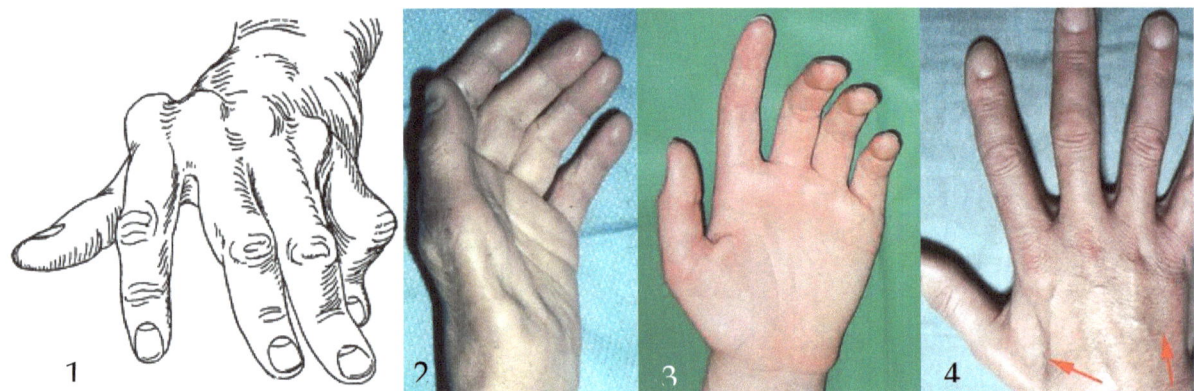

<u>MOVEMENTS</u>

Check ROM of the MCP joints, PIP joints, DIP joints. Check grip strength of the fingers.

Extension of the thumb: Affected in radial nerve lesions.

Flexion and opposition of the thumb: Affected in median nerve lesions.

Adduction of the thumb, and adduction/abduction of the other fingers: Ulnar nerve.

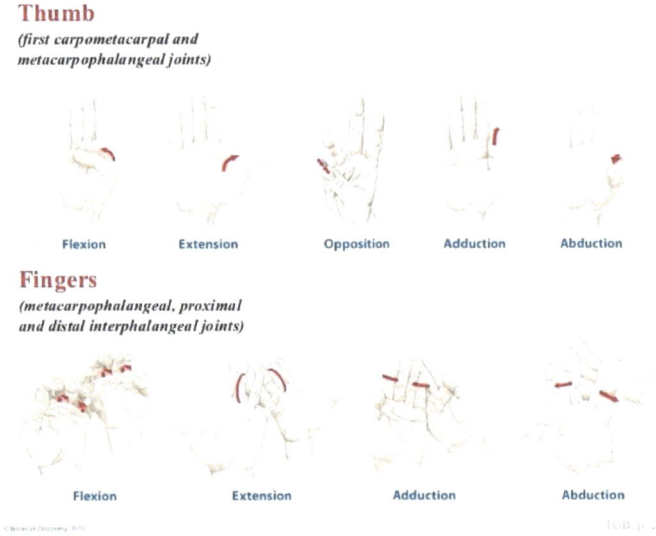

SPECIAL TESTS

Tinel's sign: Tap over the palmar aspect of the wrist on the radial side (over the median nerve area). In the presence of CTS, there may be a sensation of parasthesia ± pain in the hand (Fig. 1).
Phalen's test (reverse prayer sign): Paresthesia / pain in the median nerve distribution in the presence of carpal tunnel syndrome if the hands are held in the revere prayer position for 1 minute (Fig. 2).

Card test: Ask patient to grip a card between little and ring finger while hands vertical and examiner tries to pull away (adduction of little finger). Unable to grip in ulnar nerve lesions.

Froment sign: Patient is asked to hold a card between their thumb and index finger. The examiner then attempts to pull the object out of the subject's hands. A normal individual will be able to maintain a hold on the object without difficulty. With ulnar nerve palsy, the patient will experience difficulty maintaining a hold and will compensate by flexing the FPL (median nerve) of the thumb to maintain grip pressure causing a pinching effect (Fig. 3).

Check for wrist drop and power of extensors of the fingers: Affected in radial nerve lesions.

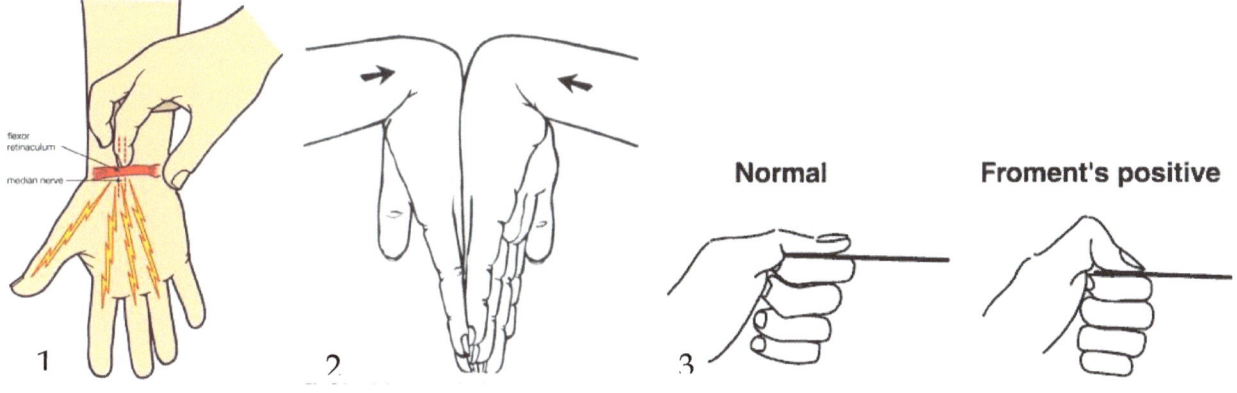

NEUROLOGICAL EXAMINATION OF UPPER LIMB

MOTOR EXAMINATION

C5: Shoulder abduction.
C6: Elbow flexion.
C7: Elbow extension & wrist extension.
C8: Wrist flexion & finger flexion (grip strength).
T1: Finger abduction / adduction.

SENSORY EXAMINATION

Always test on face or chest first.
Pain: With pin (use both blunt & sharp ends).
Light touch: Dab (don't stroke) with cotton wool.

C5: Sensations over deltoid.
C6: Over dorsal 1st web space.
C7: Tip of middle finger.
C8: Tip of little finger.
T1: Medial aspect of forearm.

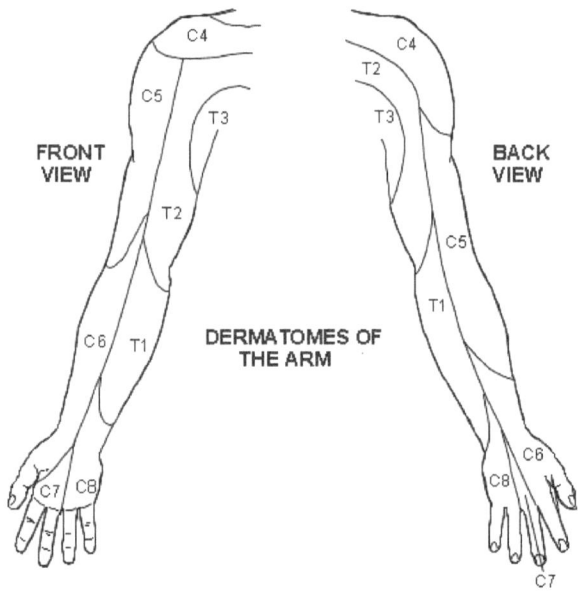

REFLEXES

Biceps reflex: C5,6.
Triceps reflex: C7,8.
Supinator reflex (Brachioradialis reflex): C6,7.

GRADING POWER

Oxford Grade	Descriptor
0	No signs of activity.
1	Flicker of activity, no movement.
2	Full active range of motion, across gravity.
3	Full active range of motion, against gravity.
4	Moderate resistance.
5	Maximal resistance.

GRADING SENSATION

Grade	Descriptor
0	Absent.
1	Altered (impaired or partial appreciation, including hyperesthesia).
2	Normal or intact.
NT	Not testable.

EXAMINATION OF HIP

ANATOMY

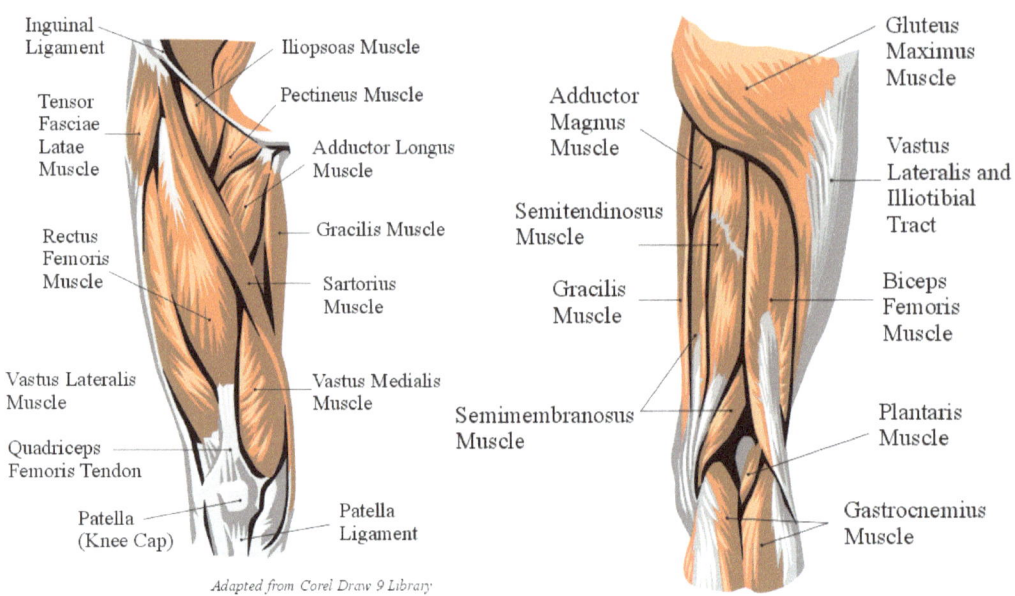

Adapted from Corel Draw 9 Library

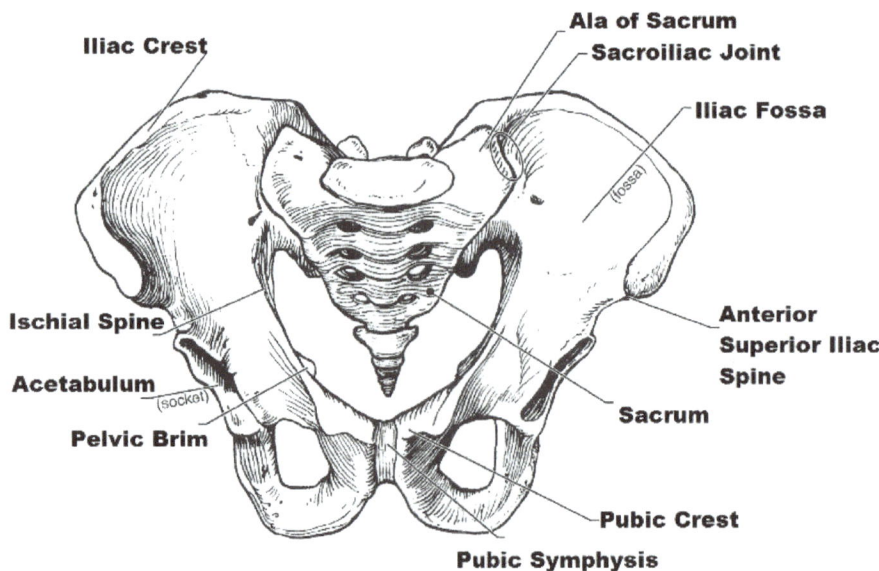

<u>INSPECTION</u>

- Examine Gait.
  A. Antalgic gait: Secondary to pain anywhere in the leg. The patient spends as little time as possible bearing weight of the affected leg. There is a fast leg swing on the contralateral leg. Patient leans towards the affected side to minimise movement of the hip.
  B. Trendelenburg gait: Caused by weakness of the abductor muscles (gluteus medius, gluteus minimus). The patient is unable to maintain hip stability, and the hip drops on the affected side. To compensate, the patient leans away from the affected side, to try and raise the hip.
  C. High stepping gait: Seen in foot drop.

- Any walking aids.
     Axillary crutches, elbow crutches, walking stick, Zimmer frame (Figs. 1-4).
- With patient facing, assess for:
     Pelvic tilt: possibly failure of adductors, short leg etc.
     Joint asymmetries, deformities: such as limb rotation, fixed flexion etc.
     Wasting of quadriceps.
- From the side:
     Lumbar lordosis: which suggests fixed flexion hip deformity.
- From behind:
     Scoliosis: primary, or may be secondary to a pelvic tilt.
     Wasting of gluteal muscles.
     Look for any signs of scars.
- Trendelenberg sign: Hold the patients hands in front of them ask them to stand on one leg at a time. Check that the hip rises on the leg that is off the floor. The pelvis on the unaffected side will drop when they stand on the affected leg (Fig. 5).

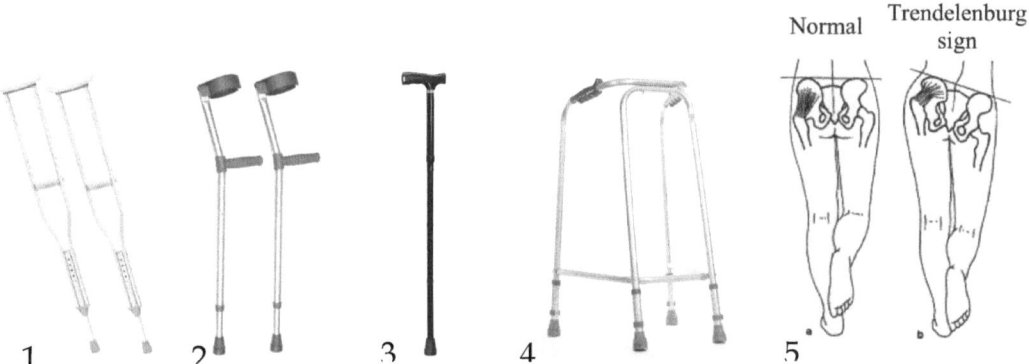

1 2 3 4 5

PALPATION

- Check whether they have any tenderness first.
- Tenderness over greater trochanter suggests trochanteric bursitis.
- Tenderness over lesser trochanter suggests iliopsoas strain.
- Tenderness over ischial tuberosity suggests hamstring strain.
- Tenderness over sacroiliac joints.
- Check for any temperature changes.

MOVEMENTS

Get the patient to lie flat on the couch. Here you can test all movements of the hip, except extension. Ask the patient to do active movements before passive. Normally both active and passive should be equal. If active movements are limited, ask the patient if this is because of pain or reduced ability to move the joint.

- Hip flexion: Flex the hip with the knee bent. Should be able to reach 120 degrees.
- Hip abduction: Stabilise the patient's pelvis by your hand on the contralateral ilium. Make sure the patient does not rotate the hip by holding the ankle. This is usually about 45 degrees.
- Hip adduction: Same as above but stabilize the ipsilateral hip first. The maximum degree of adduction is about 30 degrees.
- Internal rotation: Flex the knee to 90', and rotate the foot laterally. Normal is about 40 degrees.
- External rotation: Same as above, except rotate the foot medially. Normal is about 45 degrees.
- Extension of the hip: Ask the patient to lie prone and actively extend the hip. Normal is about 20 degrees.

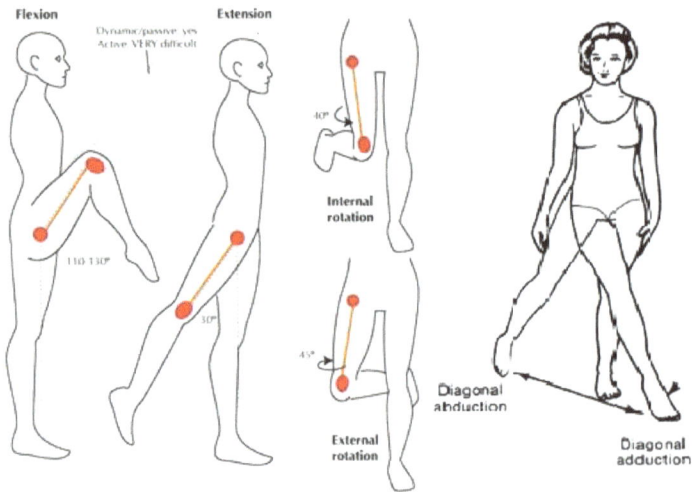

MEASUREMENTS

Patient should be supine, with pelvis squared and legs in the same posture. Compare measurements of both sides.

Apparent leg length: Measure from the xiphisternum to the medial malleolus. If there is a flexion deformity of the hip or spinal abnormalities, this will alter the 'apparent leg length', but not the true leg length.
True leg length: Measure from the anterior superior iliac spine to the medial malleolus.
Segmental length: Measure from the anterior superior iliac spine to the medial knee joint line and then from medial joint line to the medial malleolus to get the segmental lengths of the femur and tibia respectively.

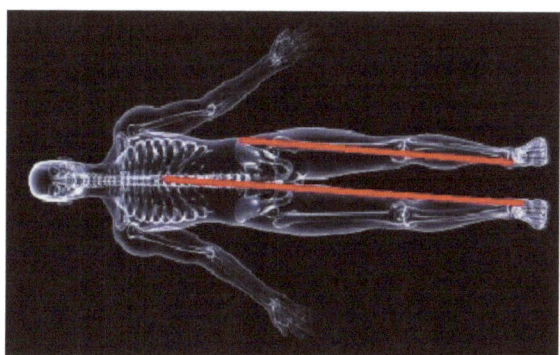

SPECIAL TESTS

- Thomas's test: Assesses for fixed flexion hip deformity. Which can occur as a result of osteoarthritis. Ask the patient to lie flat on their back. Ask the patient to flex the opposite hip to the one being tested. In a normal individual, the leg being assessed, will stay flat on the table. In fixed flexion deformity, there may be a slight raise of the leg, as the opposite one is flexed.

  You should put your left hand under the patient's lumbar spine. In a normal individual, you will feel the lumbar lordosis flatten out as the leg is raised, and the spine will press against your hand.

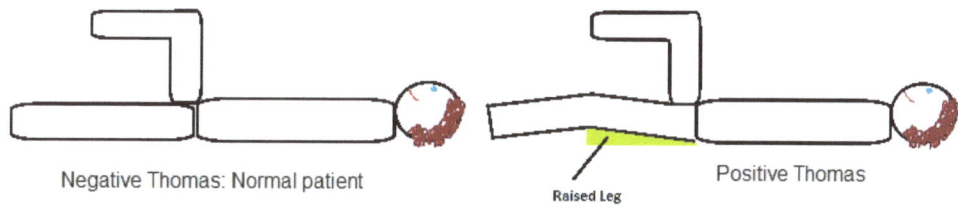

Negative Thomas: Normal patient   Raised Leg   Positive Thomas

-   Patrick test ((FABER test): The patient is positioned in supine. The leg is placed in a figure-4 position (hip flexed and abducted with the lateral ankle (malleolus) resting on the contralateral thigh just above the knee. While stabilizing the opposite side of the pelvis at the anterior superior iliac spine, an external rotation, abduction and posterior directed force is then slightly applied to the ipsilateral knee until the end range of motion (ROM) is achieved. Sacroiliac joint pain on external hip rotation is a positive Patrick's sign.

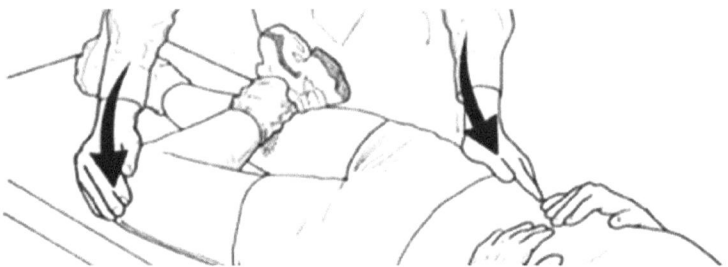

EXAMINATION OF KNEE

ANATOMY

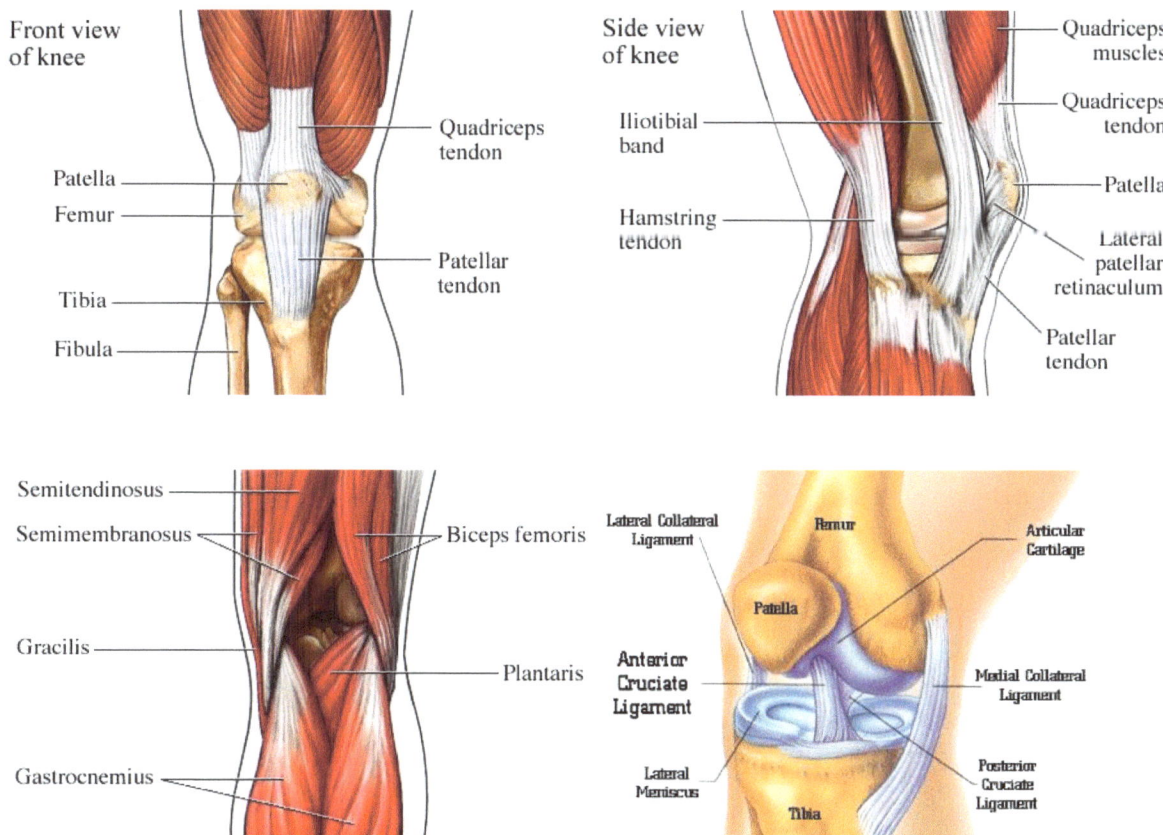

<u>INSPECTION</u>

- Gait.
- Deformities: valgus, recurvatum or varus deformity (hyperextension of the knee beyond the normal 10 degrees).
- Muscle wasting: Quadriceps bulk.
- Look for swelling: the three main causes of swollen knee are:
    Bony swellings.
    Synovial thickening.
    Fluid collection.

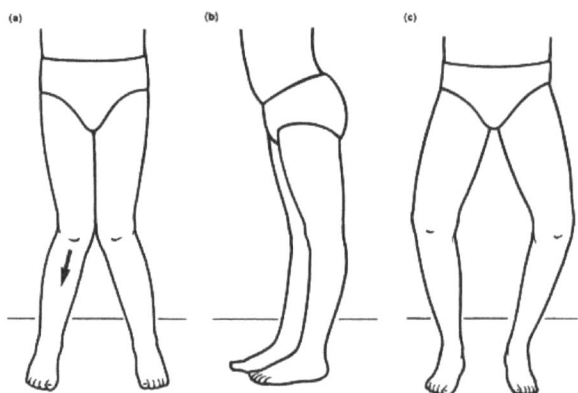

<u>PALPATION</u>

- Feel the temperature with the back of your hand. If it is warm, state there is a local rise in temperature.
- Check for tenderness at the bony points and around the knee.
- Feel the joint line: Distal to the patella, on both the medial and lateral aspects of the joint two soft triangular hollows are felt. Pressing into the superior aspect of these hollows, the joint line can be felt. Check for tenderness at the joint line.
- Feel popliteal fossa for any Baker's cyst.
- Bulge test: Can be sensitive for a small effusion.
  Put your hand about 15 cms proximal to the knee joint on the anterior part of the thigh. Then slide your hand down towards the knee. This empties the suprapatellar bursa of fluid. Keeping the first hand in place, using the other hand, press on the medial side of the knee joint to empty the medial compartment. Now all of the bursal fluid should be in the lateral compartment. Take your hand off the medial compartment, and press on the lateral compartment. You may see a bulge in the medial compartment as it fills with fluid. This shows a small effusion.
- Patella tap: Tests for larger effusions.
  Similar to the bulge test, try to empty the suprapatellar bursa. Make sure you maintain constant downwards pressure on the thigh. Now put two fingers on the patella and press firmly and briskly downwards. If fluid is present you will feel the patella move downwards (it might feel 'squishy') before hitting the underlying bone. In a normal

patient, there will be little movement of the patella, and you should not feel it hit the underlying bone.

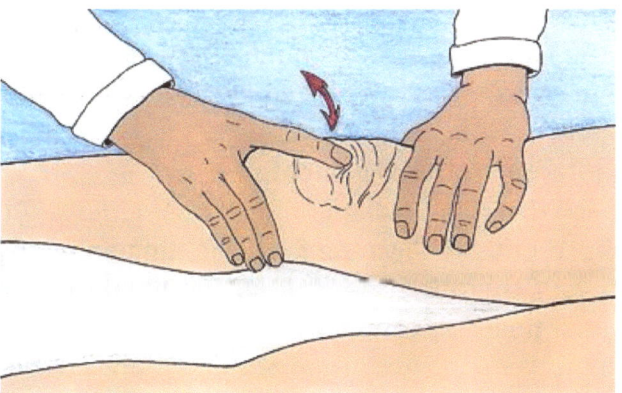

MOVEMENTS

- Extension: Ask the patient to extend their knee as far as possible. Normally about 10 degrees of hyperextension is normal.
- Flexion: Ask the patient to bring their foot to their bottom. About 150 degrees is normal.
- Compare both sides.

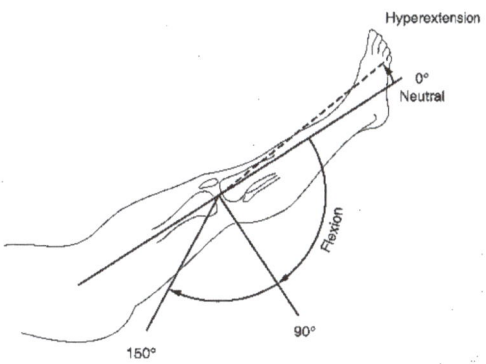

SPECIAL TESTS
- Valgus stress test: With the patient supine, extend the knee fully. Hold the ankle with one hand and the thigh with the other. Apply a valgus force at the ankle. Repeat the test with the knee in 20 degrees flexion. See if there is any abnormal opening up the joint on the stressed side. Any weakness or tear of a collateral ligament will result in a joint line that separates abnormally (Fig. 1).
- Varus stress test: With the patient supine, extend the knee fully. Hold the ankle with one hand and the thigh with the other. Apply a varus force at the ankle. Repeat the test with the knee in 20 degrees flexion. See if there is any abnormal opening up the joint on

the stressed side. Any weakness or tear of a collateral ligament will result in a joint line that separates abnormally (Fig. 2).

- Lachman's test – assesses the anterior cruciate ligament.
Flex the knee to 30 degrees. Hold the femur securely by holding the thigh firmly. Try to move the tibia forward on the femur. Normally little movement is possible. Movement >5mm suggests pathology (Fig. 3).
- Anterior drawer test: assesses the anterior cruciate ligament.
Flex both knees to 90 degrees. Check that the ankles are at the same level. Check for any sagging of tibia and correct it if present. Stabilise the foot by sitting on it. Ensure the hamstrings are relaxed. Place both your thumbs either side of the tibial tuberosity and the other fingers encircle the proximal tibia. Try to pull the tibia forward relative to the femur. Normally, there will be little movement. Abnormal anterior translation suggests an ACL pathology (Fig. 4).
- Posterior drawer test: assesses the posterior cruciate ligament. Procedure is the same as the anterior draw test, except that you push instead of pulling on the tibia.

- McMurray's test: Assesses the menisci.
With the patient supine the examiner holds the knee and palpates the joint line with one hand, thumb on one side and fingers on the other, whilst the other hand holds the sole of the foot and acts to support the limb. The knee is fully flexed. The examiner then applies a valgus stress to the knee whilst the other hand rotates the leg externally and extends the knee. Pain and/or an audible click while preforming this maneuver can indicate a torn medial meniscus. To examine the lateral meniscus the examiner repeats this process from full flexion but applies a varus stress to the knee and medial rotation to the tibia prior to extending the knee once again (Fig. 5).

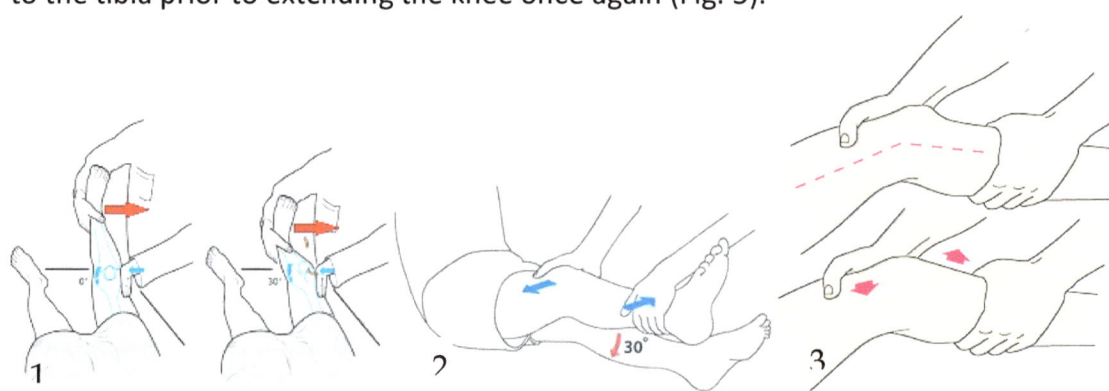

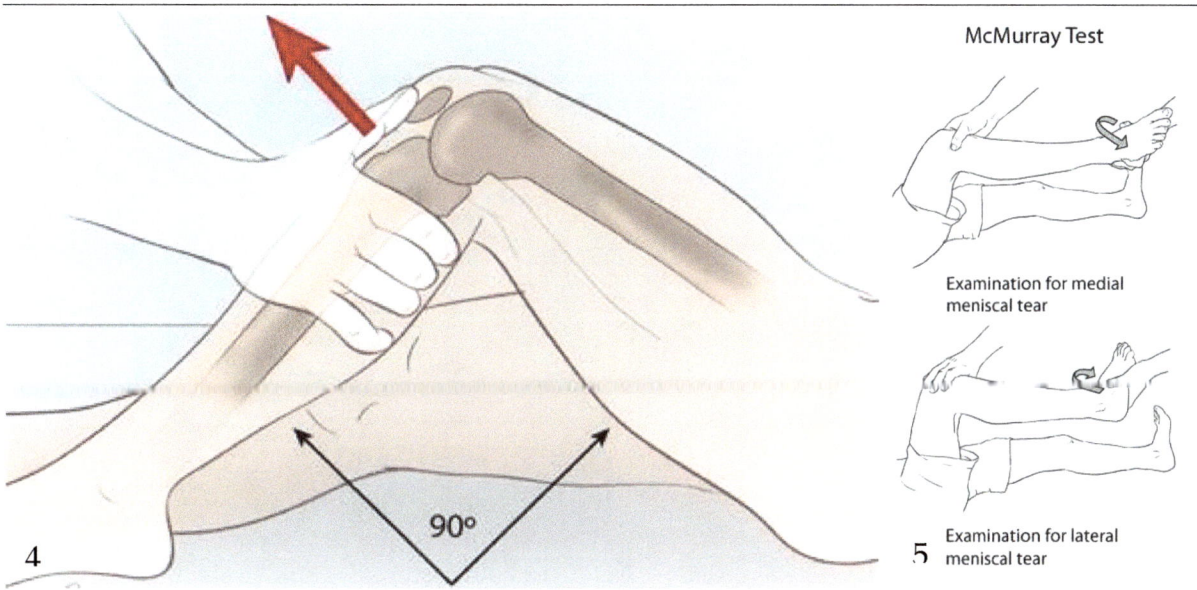

90°

4

McMurray Test

Examination for medial
meniscal tear

5   Examination for lateral
meniscal tear

EXAMINATION OF ANKLE AND FOOT

ANATOMY

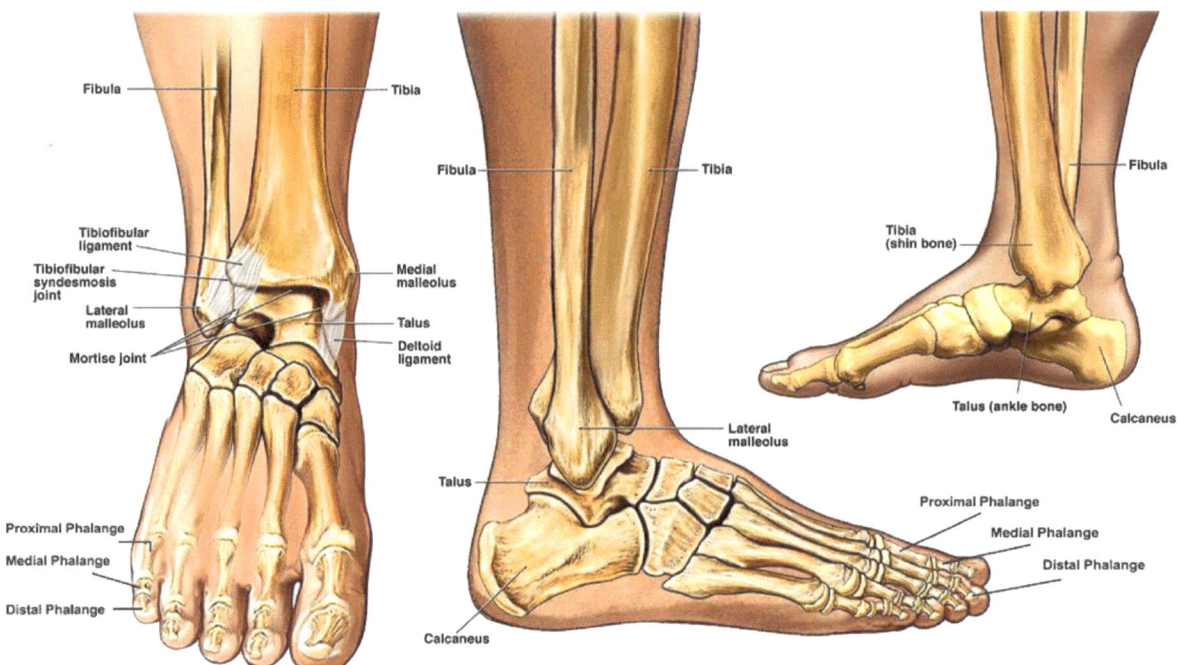

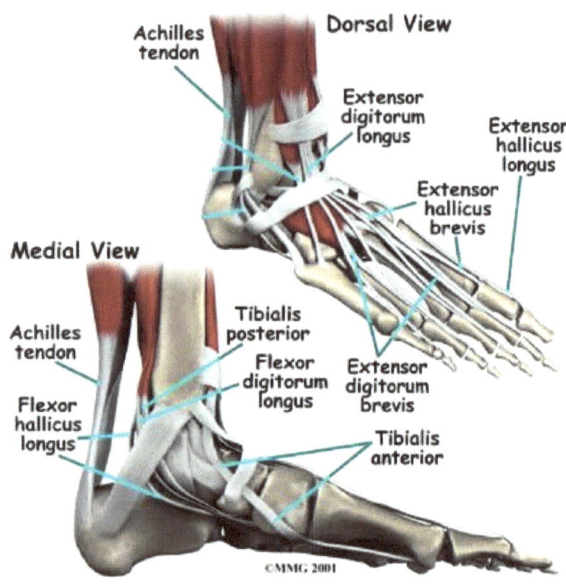

INSPECTION

- Observe the gait.
- Inspect the ankle for any obvious deformities, scars, skin colour changes, swellings, etc.

- With patient weight bearing;
- Observe the feet, comparing one with other, for symmetry.

- Look for nail changes or skin rashes such as psoriasis.
- From behind, look at the hindfoot for Achilles tendon thickening, swelling or gap.
- Look for the alignment of the toes and any evidence of hallux valgus (Fig. 1).
- Look at the arches of the feet.
  a. Flat feet: Pes planus (Fig. 2).
  b. Pes cavus: accentuated longitudinal arches that do not flatten with weight bearing (Fig. 3).
- Any swelling, clawing of toes or calluses.
- Check plantar surface for any callosities or ulcers.
- Look at the patient's footwear. Check for abnormal or asymmetrical wearing of the sole or presence of special footwear.

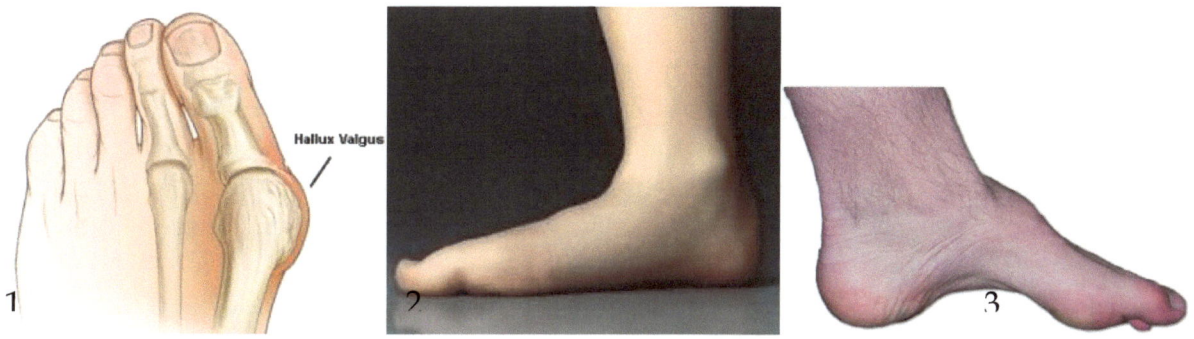

PALPATION

- Check for temperature changes: over foot and ankle.
- Check for presence of peripheral pulse.
- Gently squeeze across the MTP joints, watching patient's face for discomfort.
- Palpate the foot and ankle for tenderness.

MOVEMENTS

- Plantar flexion (movement downward) 0° to 50°.
- Dorsiflexion (movement upward) 0° to 20°.
- Inversion (turned inward) 0° to 30°.
- Eversion (turned outward) 0° to 20°.

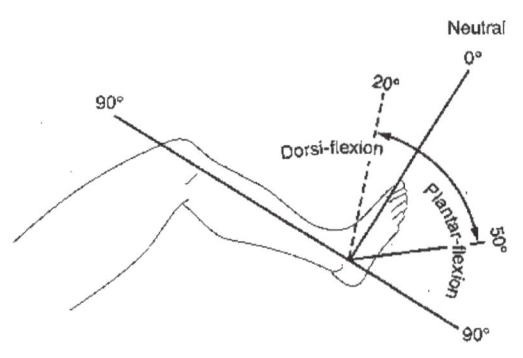 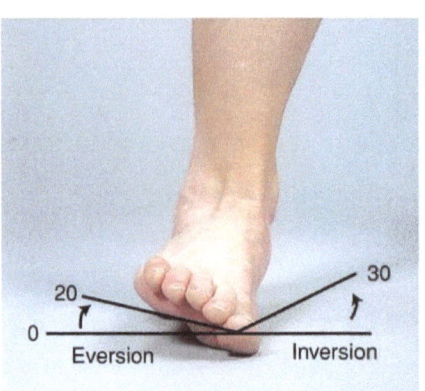

SPECIAL TESTS

- Thompson test / Simmond's test: Checks the tendoachilles for continuity. The patient lies prone with the foot over the end of the table. The examiner squeezes the calf muscles. Squeezing the calf should cause contraction of the Achilles tendon, resulting in plantar flexion. If the Achilles tendon is completely ruptured, there will not be any apparent plantar flexion (Fig 1).
- Anterior Drawer Test: Checks for anterior talofibular ligament tears.
  Patient is seated over the edge of the table with the knee bent. Examiner stabilizes the lower leg with one hand & cups the calcaneus with the forearm supporting the foot in slight plantar flexion (~ 20°) and slight inversion. The examiner then draws the calcaneus & talus anteriorly and slightly medially. A positive test is pain, anterior translation, dimple/sulcus, and/or "clunk" (Fig. 2).
- Mulder's sign: Test for Morton's neuroma. Performed with the index and thumb on the dorsal and plantar aspect of the painful intermetatarsal space. The forefoot is then compressed with the opposite hand by squeezing together the metatarsal heads. The test is positive if a painful or palpable click is felt (Fig. 3).

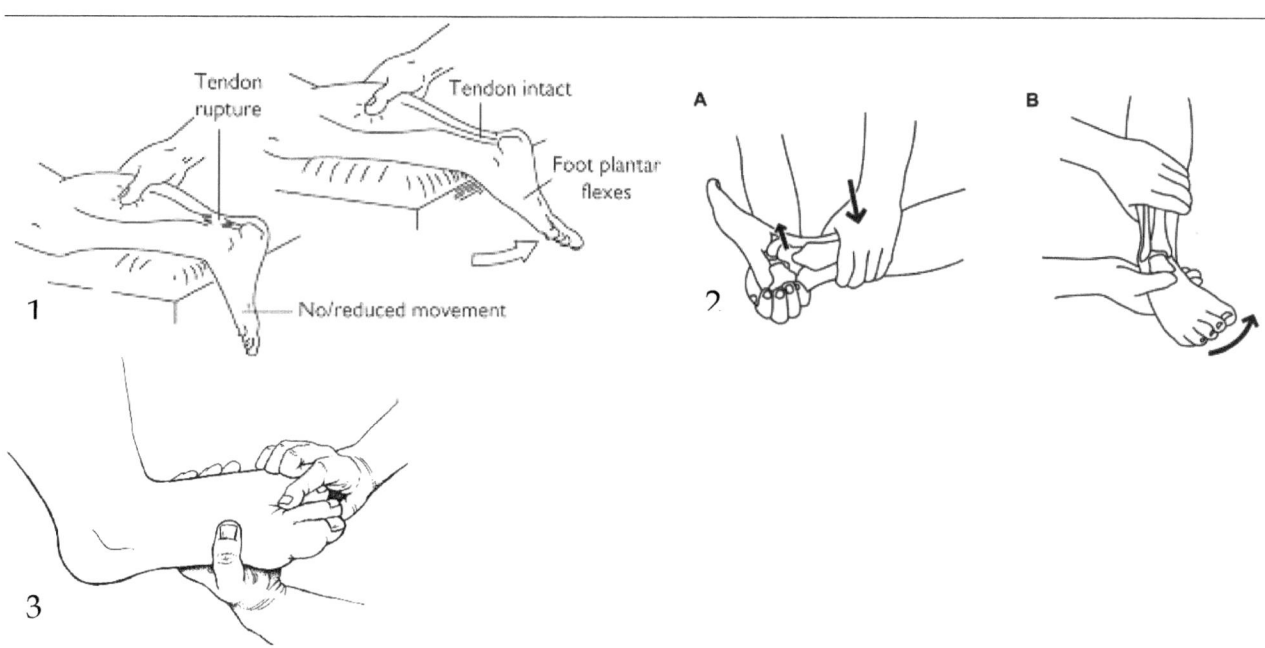

Tendon rupture

Tendon intact

Foot plantar flexes

No/reduced movement

1

A

2

B

3

NEUROLOGICAL EXAMINATION OF LOWER LIMB

MOTOR EXAMINATION

L1,2: Hip flexion.
L3: Knee extension.
L4: Ankle dorsiflexion.
L5: Toe extension.
S1: Ankle plantarflexion.

SENSORY EXAMINATION

Always test on face or chest first.
Pain: With pin (use both blunt & sharp ends).
Light touch: Dab (don't stroke) with cotton wool.

L1: Sensations over inguinal region.
L2: Over anterior thigh.
L3: Over the knee.
L4: Medial aspect of leg.
L5: Dorsum of foot.
S1: Lateral aspect of foot.
S2-5: Posterior thigh and perianal sensations.

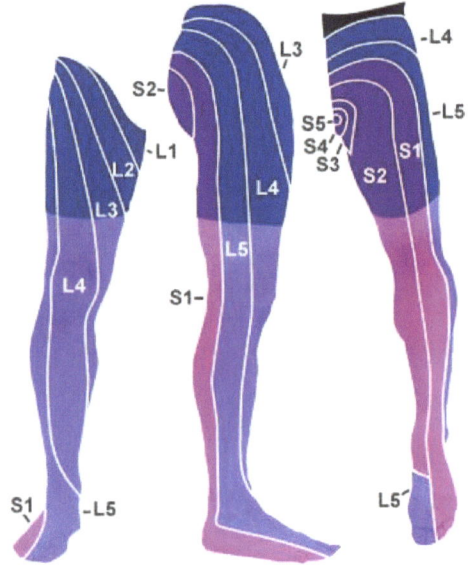

REFLEXES

Knee reflex: L3,4.
Ankle reflex: L5.
Plantar reflex: S1.

GRADING POWER

Oxford Grade	Descriptor
0	No signs of activity.
1	Flicker of activity, no movement.
2	Full active range of motion, across gravity.
3	Full active range of motion, against gravity.
4	Moderate resistance.
5	Maximal resistance.

GRADING SENSATION

Grade	Descriptor
0	Absent.
1	Altered (impaired or partial appreciation, including hyperesthesia).
2	Normal or intact.
NT	Not testable.

EXAMINATION OF SPINE
ANATOMY

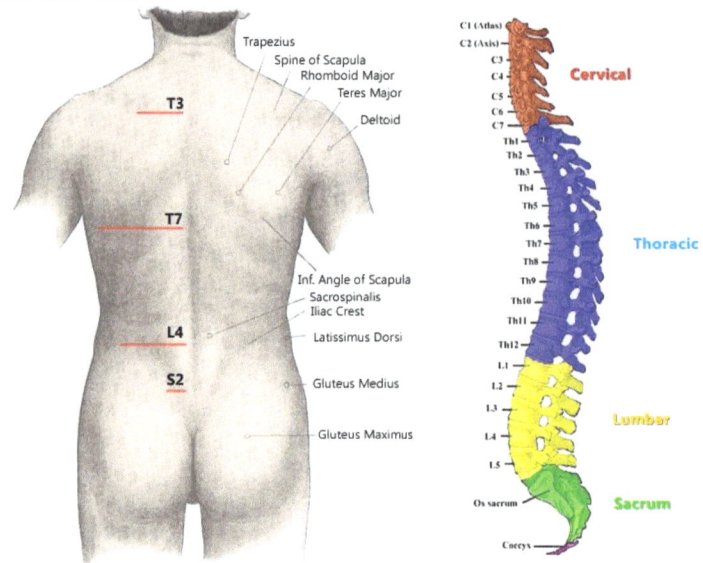

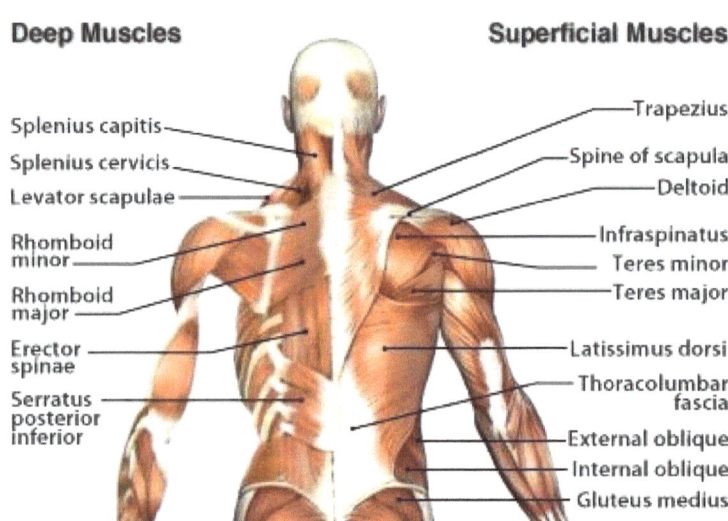

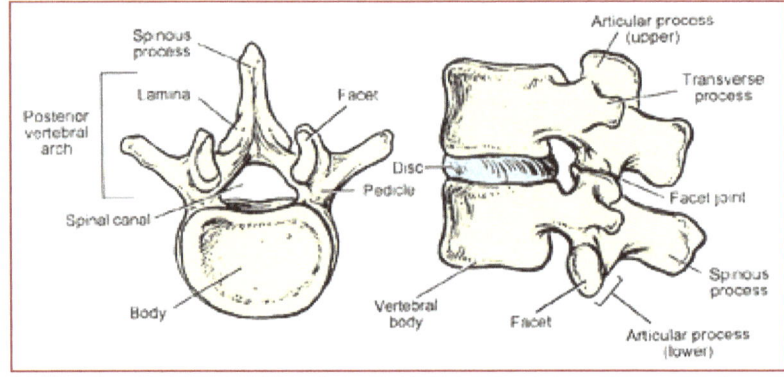

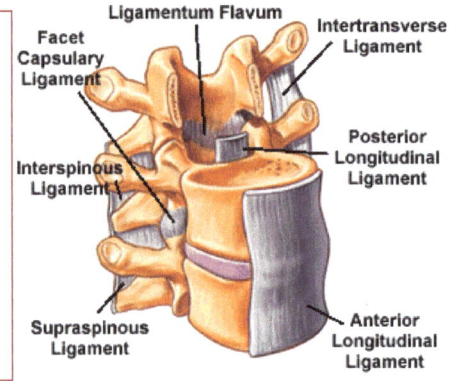

INSPECTION
- From front: Are the shoulders level?
- From side: Look for kyphosis or lordosis.
- From back: Look for any scoliosis, check shoulder level again. Look for any scars, and any wasting of the paraspinal muscles.

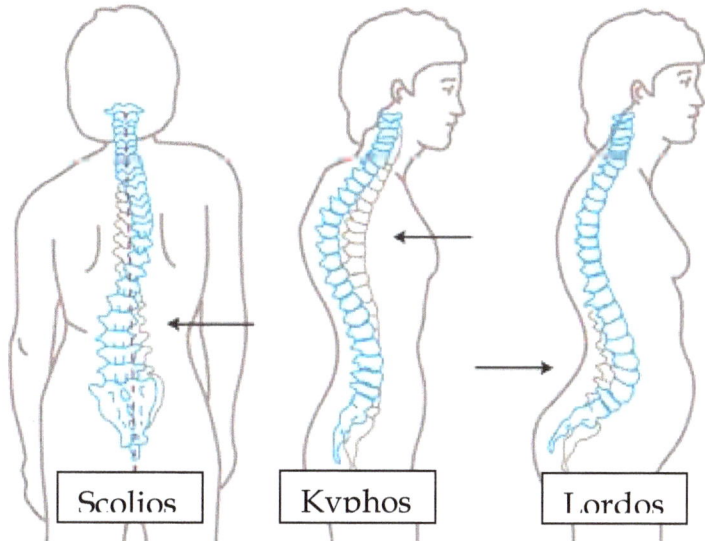

PALPATION

- Feel each vertebra in turn. Do they feel normal? Does pressing on them elicit any pain?
- Any palpable step.
- Also feel the paraspinal muscles.

MOVEMENTS

- Forward flexion:
  In cervical spine: Ask the patient to touch their chest with the chin.
  In lumbar spine: ask the patient to touch their toes, or reach as far as they can.
- Extension:
  Cervical spine: Ask the patient to look up.
  Lumbar spine: Make sure you are able to support the patient if necessary. Ask them to lean backwards, whilst keeping their hips in place.
- Lateral flexion to the right and left:
  Cervical spine: Ask the patient to try to touch their ears to the shoulder.
  Lumbar spine: Ask the patient to stand up straight with their hands down by their sides. Then ask them to lean to their left sliding the left arm towards their knee.
- Rotation to the right and left:
  Cervical spine: Ask the patient to turn their heads to look to the left and right.
  Lumbar spine: Stand behind the patient and put your hands on their hips. Then ask them to turn their back to look over their shoulder.

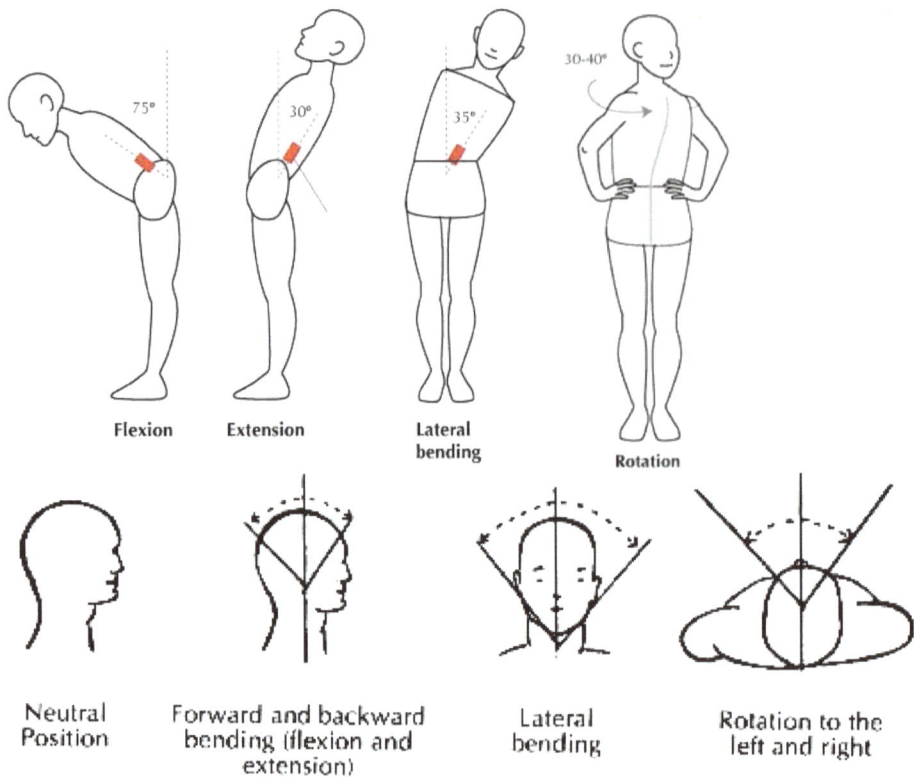

Flexion	Extension	Lateral bending	Rotation

Neutral Position	Forward and backward bending (flexion and extension)	Lateral bending	Rotation to the left and right

- Schober test: With the patient standing, find the dimples of Venus near the base of the lumbar spine. Imagine a line between these, and put a dot along this line. Then measure 10 cms above this line, and mark another dot. Then ask the patient to touch their toes (or as far as they can). Whilst in this position, re-measure this distance between your two dots. It should be >15cm. i.e. the distance should have increased by 5 cms or more.

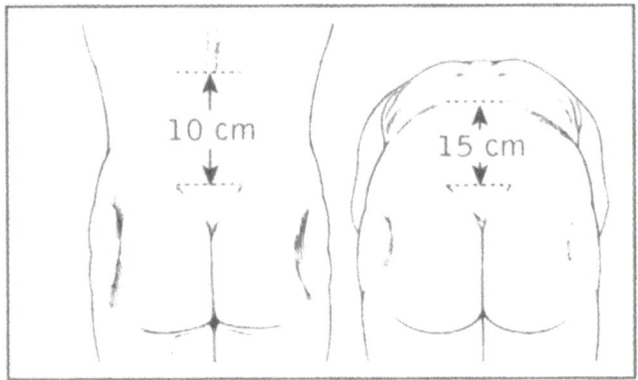

- Straight Leg Raise (SLR) test: Patient lies supine with both knees extended. Examiner stands at patient's side with distal hand cupping heel and proximal hand around patient's thigh (anteriorly) to maintain knee extension. With patient relaxed the examiner slowly raises the test leg observing for radicular pain (Fig. 1).
- Lasegue's test: Do the SLR test. Once patient complains of pain, the examiner slowly lowers the leg until the pain or tightness just resolves, and then dorsiflexes the ankle. The pain will be reproduced in a positive test (Fig.1 inset).
- Bowstring test: Subject begins supine with legs extended. Examiner performs a passive straight leg raise on the involved side. If radiating pain is reported, the examiner then flexes the patient's knee until symptoms are reduced. The examiner then applies pressure to the popliteal area in attempt to reproduce the radicular pain. Positive test is reproduction of radicular pain with popliteal compression (Fig. 2).

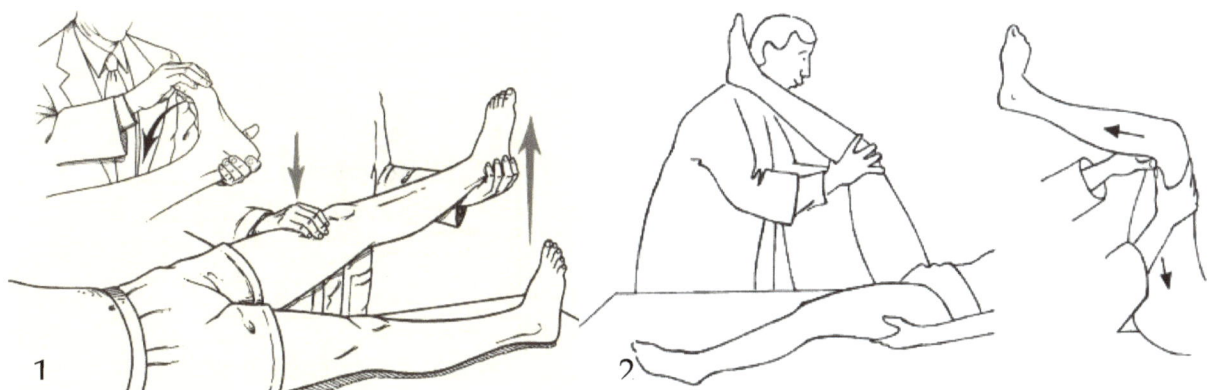

NEUROLOGICAL EXAMINATION
- Assess tone of the limbs.
- Check the dermatomes and myotomes.
- Perform the reflexes.

GALS EXAMINATION

This stands for Gait, Arms, Legs, Spine.

The exam is a quick way of screening for musculoskeletal dysfunction. Most of the exam can be done without actually having to touch the patient, just ask them to copy your movements. It is not a diagnostic examination, but basically a screening technique to asses if there may be underlying pathology that needs further investigation.

GAIT

- Does the patient need a walking aid?
- Check symmetry.
- How easily is the patient able to stand up and sit down in a chair?
- Is there varus or valgus deformity?
- Are the feet abnormally inverted / everted?
- Are they generally unsteady (especially when turning)?
- Look at posture: Look at the normal spinal curvature and see if there are any abnormalities.
- Is the patient able to turn quickly?

ARMS

HANDS

- Quick inspection for any obvious abnormalities and deformities.
- Ask the patient to make the prayer sign. This tests MCP, PIP and DIP extension & extension of the wrist.
- Ask them to make the inverted prayer sign.
- Ask the patient to make a fist. Assess grip.
- Assess pinch: Check all fingers can oppose, and then test pinch strength.
- Squeeze the MCP joints: crude test for inflammatory arthritis.
- Check the tendon sheaths for thickening and trigger finger.

ELBOWS

- Quick inspection for any obvious abnormalities.
- Check for full extension.
- Test if the patient can touch their ipsilateral shoulders (flexion).
- Test for pronation and supination.

SHOULDER

- Quick inspection for any obvious abnormalities.
- Check abduction, flexion, internal rotation and external rotation.
- Abduction and external rotation can be examined together by asking the patient to put their hands on the back of their head.

LEGS

HIPS
- Patient supine on bed.
- Check tenderness and ROM.

KNEES
- Look for swelling and, and check for effusions by patellar tap.
- Look at quadriceps bulk.
- Look for varus and valgus deformity.

FOOT AND ANKI F
- Inspect the sole of the foot for callosities.
- Look for abnormal separation of the toes.
- Squeeze the MTP joints: Screening for inflammatory arthritis.
- Check the foot arches.

SPINE
- Examine from the front, side and back.
- Observe, and check for any gross abnormalities, normal spinal curvature, and shoulder height.
- Feel down the length of the spine feeling the spinous processes & paraspinal muscles.
- Check for ROM at the cervical and lumbar spines.

NEONATAL ORTHOPAEDIC SCREENING

All new born babies have to be examined for hip dysplasias, limb abnormalities and spinal dysraphism.

- Hip dysplasia:
A. Ortolani test: The examiner's hands are placed over the child's knees with his/her thumbs on the medial thigh and the fingers placing a gentle upward stress on the lateral thigh and greater trochanter area. With slow abduction, a dislocated and reducible hip will reduce with a described palpable "clunk."

B. Barlow Maneuver: Guide the hips into mild adduction and applying a slight forward pressure with the thumb. If the hip is unstable, the femoral head will slip over the posterior rim of the acetabulum, again producing a palpable sensation of subluxation or dislocation.

The degree of instability can be described as:

1. Dislocated and reducible (+ Ortolani).

2. Dislocated and irreducible (- Ortolani).

3. Dislocatable (+ Barlow).

4. Subluxed (a hip with mild instability or laxity with a – Barlow maneuver).

After 2-3 months of age, the Barlow and Ortolani tests are less reproducible. At this age the following features may be seen.
   A. Galeazzi sign: Unilateral dysplasia presenting as asymmetric shortening on the side of the dislocation.
   B. Tight hip adductors/decreased hip abduction.
   C. Asymmetric thigh or gluteal folds.

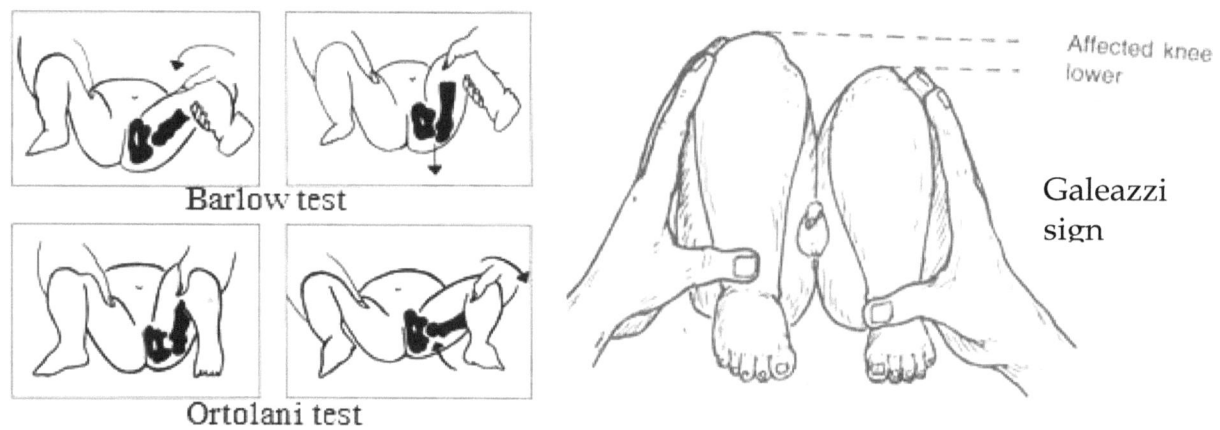

Barlow test

Ortolani test

Affected knee lower

Galeazzi sign

- Spinal dysraphism: Look for any midline dimple, subcutaneous mass, nevus, tuft of hair or altered skin pigmentation.

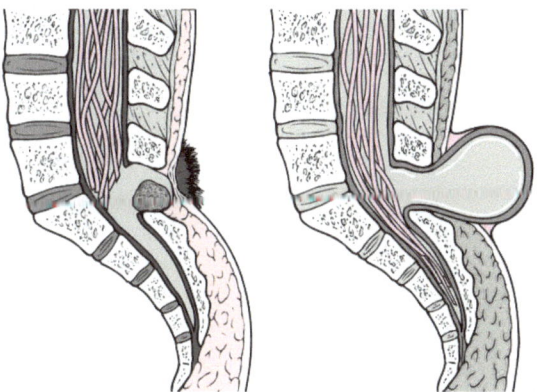

EXAMINATION OF AN ULCER
INSPECTION

- Site.
- Size.
- Shape.
- Number.
- Margin: line of demarcation between normal and abnormal.
    Well demarcated.
    Not demarcated.
- Floor: the exposed part of an ulcer.
    Slough: Moist dead tissue.
    Scab: Dry dead tissue.
    Unhealthy granulation tissue.
    Healthy granulation tissue.
    Subcutaneous fat.
    Muscle/tendons.
    Bone.
- Edge: the part between the margin and the floor of an ulcer.
    Slopping: Healing ulcer.
    Punched out: Decubitus ulcer/Gummatous ulcer.
    Undermined: Tuberculous ulcer.
    Raised / Beaded: Basal cell carcinoma.
    Rolled out / everted: Squamous cell carcinoma.
- Discharge: Note the colour, amount & smell.
    Serous: Healing ulcer.
    Sanguineous (blood stained): Malignant/Chronic.
    Purulent: Bacterial infection.
    Greenish: Pseudomonas infection.
    Yellowish: Sulphur granules (Actinomycosis).

PALPATION
- Local rise of temperature & tenderness.
- Exact dimensions: Depth.
- Induration (thickening) of edge: In chronic ulcer and in malignancy.
- Base: The structure on which the ulcer rests. Fixity to underlying structures.
- Bleeding on touch is a feature of malignant / chronic ulcer.

EXAMINATION OF THE SURROUNDING AREA OF AN ULCER

- Skin, adjacent joint, regional lymph nodes.
- Arterial pulse, varicose veins, neurological deficits, gait of the patient.

EXAMINATION OF A LUMP

INSPECTION

-   Site.
-   Number.
-   Size.
-   Shape.
-   Surrounding skin.
-   Surface: Smooth vs. rough vs. indurated.
-   Skin, scars.
-   Edge: Clear vs. poorly defined.
-   Trans illumination, if applicable.

PALPATION

-   Temperature: Feel with back of fingers on surface and surroundings.
-   Tenderness.
-   Consistency: Soft, firm or hard.
-   Mobility and attachment: Move lump in two directions, right-angled to each other. Then repeat exam when muscle contracted.
    Bone: Immobile.
    Muscle: Contraction reduces lump mobility.
    Subcutaneous: Skin can move over lump.
    Skin: Moves with skin.
-   Pulsatile: Assess with 2 fingers on mass.
    Transmitted pulsation: Both fingers pushed same direction.
    Expansile: Fingers diverge (especially for AAA).
-   Fluctuation: Assess by placing 2 fingers in "peace sign" on either edge of lump, then tapping lump center with index finger of other hand: fluctuant lump will displace peace sign fingers.
-   Irreducible.
-   Compressible: Mass decreases with pressure, but reappears immediately upon release.
-   Reducible: Mass reappears only on cough, etc.
-   Regional lymph nodes around mass.

PERCUSSION AND AUSCULTATION

-   Percussion: Dull / resonant.
-   Auscultation: Bruit.

INDEX

www.ingramcontent.com/pod-product-compliance
Lightning Source LLC
Chambersburg PA
CBHW050806180526
45159CB00004B/1570